ANTI-CANCER
PLANT-BASED DIET
COOKBOOK
FOR
WOMEN

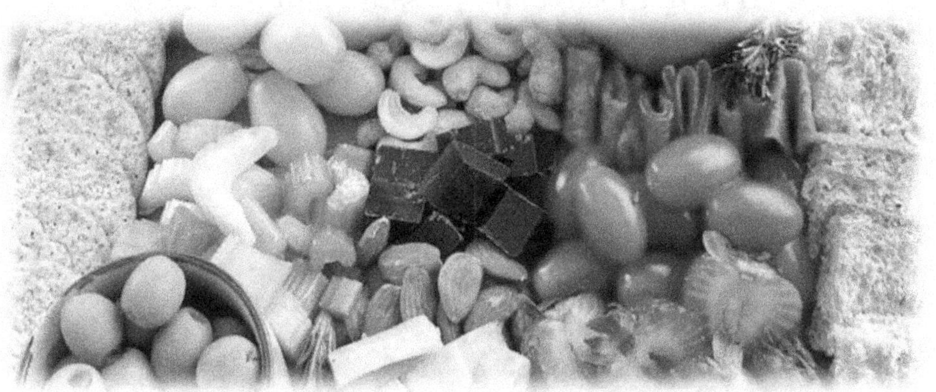

Quick, easy and delectable whole food Comforting Recipes to Fight, combat, reverse and nourish Your Body during and after cancer

KIMBERLY WRIGHT

COPYRIGHT

All rights reserved. No part of this book may be reproduced in any form or by any electronic or mechanical means, including information storage and retrieval systems, without permission in writing from the publisher, except by a reviewer who may quote brief passages in a review.

Copyright © 2024 by [**Kimberly wright**]

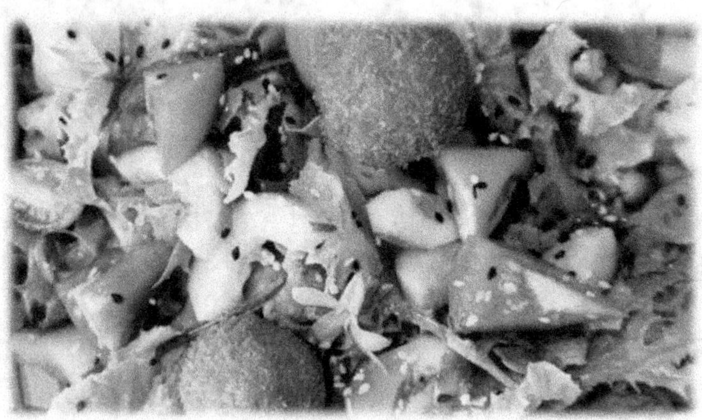

Dear Beautiful Souls,

Your thoughts and views are priceless treasures in our quest to create content that resonates with you. If this book brought you a smile or peace, we urge you to express your thoughts through a passionate review. Your input is a priceless gift that allows us to improve our materials and make them even more pleasurable for other survivors and enthusiasts alike.

In gratitude for your kindness,

[Kimberly Wright]

TABLE OF CONTENTS

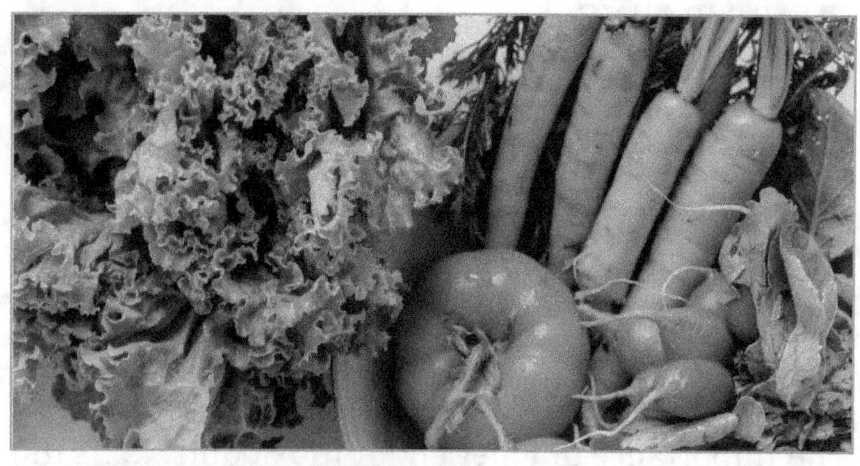

Hello, lovely individuals on this magnificent adventure we call life! If you've made it here, it means you're ready to start on a transforming odyssey—a voyage beyond ordinary life, a path to robust health, and a book that's more than merely recipes. The "Anti-Cancer Plant-Based Diet Cookbook for Women" is here!

Let us dive into the core of life: health. We're not just talking about a cookbook; we're revealing a road map to vitality, a treasure trove of delicious meals that not only tickle your taste buds but also act as potent weapons against cancer's horrific antagonist.

Cancer is that awful term that sends shivers down the spines of our collective brain. But what if I told you that within these pages lies a key, a powerful ally against this adversary? The first step in defeating cancer is to understand it. It's not simply renegade cells; it's a war within, and nutrition is crucial.

Friends, let's communicate with facts. Did you know that, according to the World Health Organization, dietary modifications can prevent almost one-third of cancer cases? The most critical lifestyle modification is controlling what you put on your plate. Food is more than simply fuel—it is a healer and a shield. Let's go right to the point: the revolution centered around plants. Imagine consuming a meal abundant in the brilliant colors of the natural world, a culinary symphony composed by Mother Earth herself. Eating plant-based is a time-tested, science-backed perception that follows the adage "Let thy food be thy medicine." It is not a fad.

Settle into your chairs, for here is the last twist: Studies regularly demonstrate that plant-based diets dramatically lower the incidence of lung, breast, prostate, and colon cancers, among other malignancies. It's the armor your body needs to fight cancer; it's not a miracle treatment.

Let me tell you a story that bridges the gap between triumph and adversity, a narrative that is a light of hope. It is a tale of a fighter and survivor who outwitted and outlasted cancer. Meet Sarah, a warrior who defeated cancer by dancing with it. Sarah Andrew has an infectious smile who effortlessly wins people over without her even trying. Sarah flourished rather than merely endure, thanks to the recipes you'll find in this book. Picture yourself enjoying foods that entice your palate and provide your cells energy. This cookbook can help you achieve the same results as it did for Sarah.

Here is a call to action as much as a cookbook. Imagine the smell of spices filling your kitchen as you turn the pages, the sound of healthful foods sizzling in your pan, and the satisfaction from nourishing your body with each meal. Simple, quick, and delicious—because improving your health should be a joy rather than a job.

My dearest one, are you prepared to fight, reverse, and support your body throughout and after cancer treatment? Accept a voyage full of taste, energy, and tenacity. Accept the offering of the "Anti-Cancer Plant-Based Diet Cookbook for Women." Your body is your temple; therefore, let's both paint it in the brilliant colors of health.

Flip the page and let the recovery commence.

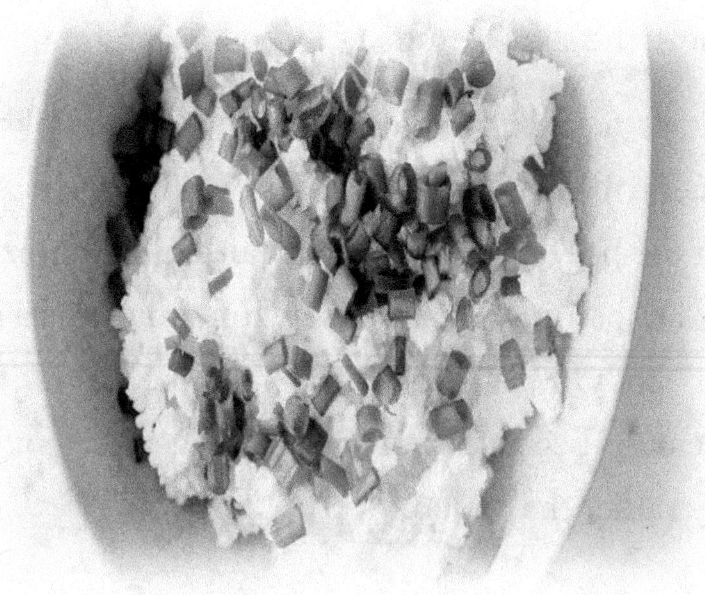

CHAPTER ONE

The Power of Eating Right to Fight Cancer

A disease known as cancer occurs when some cells in the body multiply out of control and invade other parts of the human body. With billions of cells making up the human body, cancer may begin practically anywhere. Human cells typically grow to create new cells as needed by the body by increasing and multiplying. New cells replace old ones when they die due to aging or injury.

This controlled mechanism can occasionally malfunction, causing damaged or aberrant cells to increase and expand when they shouldn't. Tumors are lumps of tissue that can be formed by these cells. Cancerous or benign tumors can both occur.

Malignant tumors can metastasize or spread into surrounding tissues and generate new tumors by traveling to far-off regions of the body. Malignant tumors are another term for cancerous tumors.

Blood malignancies, including leukemias, often do not develop into solid tumors, but many cancers do.

Benign tumors do not penetrate or spread to tissue nearby. Benign tumors seldom come back after removal, while malignant ones occasionally do. However, benign tumors can sometimes grow to be rather enormous. Some, like benign brain tumors, are potentially fatal or produce severe symptoms.

How Does Cancer Develop?

Cancer is a hereditary disease, indicating that alterations to the genes that regulate our cells' growth and division cause cancer.

Cancer-causing genetic alterations may result from:

- Mistakes made during cell division.
- Of damage to DNA resulting from exposure to dangerous environmental elements, such as UV radiation from the sun and toxins in cigarette smoke.
- Our parents passed these on to us.

Usually, damaged DNA cells are eliminated by the body before they become malignant. However, the body's capacity to do so decreases as we age, contributing to the increased risk of cancer in later life.

A different mix of genetic alterations causes everybody's cancer. There will be further alterations as the cancer spreads. Various cells within the same tumor may exhibit distinct genetic alterations.

Proto-oncogenes, tumor suppressor genes, and DNA repair genes are the three primary gene categories typically impacted by genetic alterations leading to cancer. These alterations are occasionally referred to as cancer "drivers."

Proto-oncogenes play a role in the proper division and development of cells. On the other hand, these genes may become cancer-causing genes (also known as oncogenes), allowing cells to proliferate and survive when they shouldn't be changing in specific ways or becoming more active than usual.

Additionally, tumor suppressor genes regulate the division and development of cells. Certain tumor suppressor gene mutations can cause uncontrollably dividing cells.

Genes that repair damaged DNA are known as DNA repair genes. Mutations in these genes frequently lead to further modifications in other genes and chromosomal abnormalities, such as duplications and deletions of chromosomal segments in the cells. When combined, these alterations have the potential to make the cells malignant.

Scientists have discovered that specific mutations are frequently present in various cancer forms as they continue to understand more about the molecular alterations that cause cancer. Nowadays, many cancer therapies focus on the gene abnormalities that cause cancer. Anybody with cancer with the targeted mutation can utilize some of these therapies, regardless of the disease's initial growth origin.

When Cancer Spreads

Metastatic cancer is a kind of cancer that has spread to various parts of the body from its original site. Metastasis is the process by which cancer cells move to different areas of the body.

The initial, or primary, cancer and metastatic cancer have the same name and kind of cancer cells. For instance, breast cancer that spreads to the lung and develops into a tumor is called metastatic breast cancer, not lung cancer.

Metastatic cancer cells often appear like the initial cancer cells under a microscope. Furthermore, some molecular characteristics, such as specific chromosomal alterations, are typically shared by the original and metastatic cancer cells.

In certain circumstances, treatment may help patients with metastatic cancer survive longer. In other instances, stopping the disease's spread or reducing its symptoms are the main objectives of treatment for metastatic cancer. Most cancer deaths are due to metastatic illness, and metastatic tumors can seriously impair a person's ability to operate.

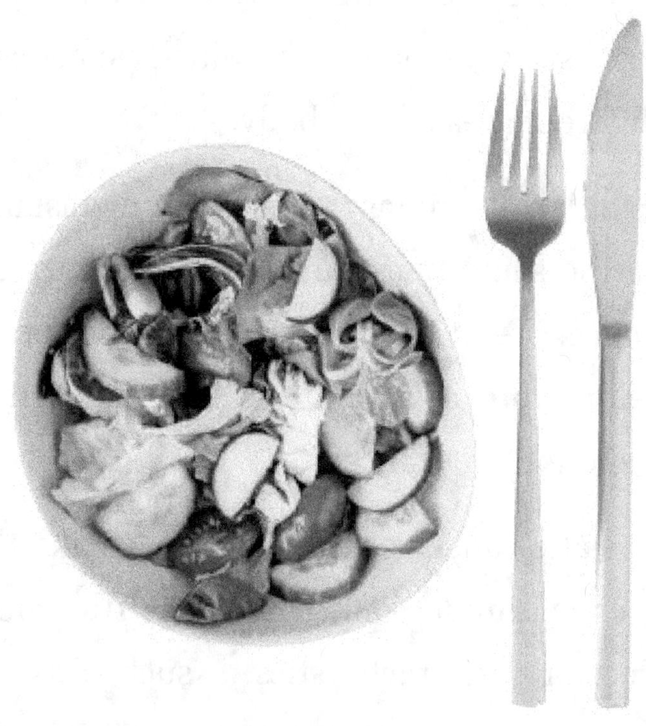

CHAPTER TWO

Types of Cancer

Cancer comes in more than a hundred varieties. The organs or tissues where tumors originate are typically used for naming different types of cancer. For instance, brain cancer begins in the brain, but lung cancer starts in the lung. Cancers can also be classified according to the kind of cell that gave rise to them, such as squamous or epithelial cells.

The following are some forms of malignancies that start in specific cell types:

Here are some categories of cancers that begin in specific types of cells:

Carcinoma

Carcinomas are the most common type of cancer. They are formed by epithelial cells, which are the cells that cover the inside and outside surfaces of the body. When viewed under a microscope, many types of epithelial cells often have a column-like shape.

Carcinomas that begin in different epithelial cell types have specific names:

Adenocarcinoma is a cancer in epithelial cells that produce fluids or mucus. Tissues with this type of epithelial cell are sometimes called glandular tissues. Most cancers of the breast, colon, and prostate are adenocarcinomas.

Basal cell carcinoma is a cancer that begins in the lower or basal (base) layer of the epidermis, which is a person's outer layer of skin.

Squamous cell carcinoma is a cancer that forms in squamous cells, which are epithelial cells that lie just beneath the skin's outer surface. Squamous cells also line many other organs, including the stomach, intestines, lungs, bladder, and kidneys. Squamous cells look flat, like fish scales, when viewed under a microscope. Squamous cell carcinomas are sometimes called epidermoid carcinomas.

Lymphoma

Cancer that starts in lymphocytes is called lymphoblast's (T cells or B cells). These are immune system-fighting white blood cells that combat illness. Abnormal lymphocytes accumulate in lymphoma lymph nodes, lymph arteries, and other bodily organs.

Two primary forms of lymphoma exist:

Hodgkin lymphoma: Individuals with this illness have Reed-Sternberg cells, which are aberrant lymphocytes. Usually, B cells give rise to these cells.

Non-Hodgkin lymphoma is a broad category of malignancies that originate in the lymph nodes. B cells or T cells can give rise to malignancies, which can develop swiftly or slowly.

Multiple Myeloma

Another kind of immune cell called a plasma cell is the source of multiple myeloma. Myeloma cells, which are aberrant plasma cells, accumulate in the bone marrow and develop into tumors in bones throughout the body. Kahler disease and plasma cell myeloma are other names for multiple myeloma.

Melanoma

Cancer that starts in cells that develop into melanocytes, which are specialized cells that produce melanin, the pigment responsible for skin color, is known as melanoma. Although melanomas most commonly occur on the skin, they can also develop in other pigmented tissues, such as the eye.

Spinal cord and brain tumors

Tumors of the brain and spinal cord can be of several kinds. The basis for their names is the cellular type in which these tumors originated and the location of the tumor's initial formation inside the central nervous system. For instance, astrocytes, which are star-shaped brain cells that support nerve cells' health, are an astrocytic tumor's starting point. Brain tumors can be benign (not cancer) or malignant (cancer).

A cancer diagnosis is frequently related to environmental factors, lifestyle decisions, or family medical history. Furthermore, although your surroundings and family history are beyond your control, you can influence healthy lifestyle choices, including maintaining a healthy weight, exercising frequently, eating a balanced diet, and giving up smoking if you smoke often.

Although each person's risk factors are unique, it's crucial to understand that you may take steps to reduce your risk.

Understanding your risk factors and learning how to modify them is crucial, as estimated 282,500 women are expected to die from cancer in 2017, and approximately 852,630 women are expected to receive a cancer diagnosis, according to estimates published in the American Cancer Society (ACS) "Cancer Facts and Figures 2017" report.

Reapplying sunscreen after spending time outside can help prevent skin cancer, among other basic preventative measures. Generally, I recommend discussing your risk factors based on your lifestyle and family history with your doctor. Understanding your limitations might assist you in creating a tailored strategy that includes what tests you would need to have (and when), what dietary adjustments could be beneficial, and other things. "Changing one item could benefit one individual but not necessarily help another.

Find out more about the factors that might raise your chance of developing any of the top five malignancies that affect women, as well as some preventative measures.

Breast Cancer

Thirty percent of female cancer diagnoses and fourteen percent of the anticipated 282,500 female cancer deaths in 2017 are expected to be related to breast cancer. The risk of breast cancer in women is 1 in 8.

Although there isn't a single, effective method to avoid breast cancer, and many risk factors are beyond your control, knowing the most prevalent risk factors below will help you manage the ones that are.

As a female, Women are around 100 times more likely than males to develop breast cancer.

Age: 55 years of age or older accounts for two out of every three cases of invasive breast cancer in women.

Family history: If your mother, sister, or daughter has ever had breast cancer, your risk is doubled. If two immediate family members have had it, your risk is quadrupled. Different screening recommendations may apply depending on your family history, so discuss your options with your doctor.

Between 5 and 10 percent of breast cancers are believed to be caused by specific inherited gene abnormalities; the most often associated mutations to the illness are BRCA1 and BRCA2.

Color: African-American women are more likely to die from breast cancer than white women, primarily because of the possibility that their tumors would develop more quickly and manifest at an advanced stage.

Dense breast tissue: Having more fibrous and glandular tissue rather than fatty tissue owing to age, menopausal status, certain medicines, pregnancy, and genetics can double the risk of breast cancer and make detecting early malignancies on a mammogram more difficult.

Previous chest radiation therapy: Women previously treated for another cancer are at an increased risk of getting breast cancer, especially if the treatment was received when their breasts were still growing.

A larger than usual number of menstrual cycles (beginning of menstruation before the age of 12, start of menopause after the age of 55) increases risk marginally.

No pregnancies or late first pregnancy (beyond 30) boosts overall risk little, while pregnancy may increase the chance of specific breast cancer subtypes, such as triple-negative disease.

Birth control pills: The level of risk appears to return to normal ten years after a woman discontinues use. Past usage of diethylstilbestrol (DES), a medication initially used to prevent miscarriage, somewhat enhances the risk of breast cancer.

Avoiding post-menopausal hormone therapy reduces your chance of breast cancer.

Breast cancer risk may be somewhat increased if you do not breastfeed.

Being overweight (especially after menopause) raises the risk. Working with a nutritionist to determine how to change your diet may assist you in losing weight and lowering your risk. Furthermore, losing weight might lessen the quantity of estrogen; breast cancer feeds on estrogen, and this hormone is more abundant in obese persons.

Lack of exercise has been related to an increased risk of breast cancer, so if you're sedentary, try to move more. Exercise is always a good idea.

Excessive drinking According to the American Cancer Society, women who drink one daily have a slightly higher risk of breast cancer than nondrinkers. In contrast, women who drink two to three drinks daily have a 20% greater chance of having the illness.

Red meat eating has also been linked to breast cancer. However, doctors aren't sure if it may trigger the illness. If you're in danger, try eating more white meat and seafood.

In 2017, lung and bronchus malignancies were predicted to account for 12% of female cancer diagnoses and 25% of female cancer fatalities. A woman's chances of developing lung cancer are 1 in 17.

A look at the percentages of fatalities among patients diagnosed with this type of cancer demonstrates how lethal it is. Though breast cancer is far more common in women than lung cancer, the latter causes far more fatalities. Most startling is our potential to reduce those numbers: 80 percent of all lung cancers in women (and 90 percent in males) could be averted if individuals did not smoke. According to the Centers for Disease Control and Prevention, smokers are 15 to 30 times more likely than non-smokers to develop or die from lung cancer. Family history also plays a vital part.

Other risk factors for lung cancer include exposure to:

Secondhand smoke

Radon gas

Arsenic (either breathed or in drinking water)

Asbestos

Emissions from diesel engines

Air pollution

Aside from exercising and eating a healthy diet, minimizing your alcohol intake can help lessen your risk of lung cancer. And even if you are now a former smoker, if you smoked a pack of cigarettes a day for 30 years, guidelines recommend that you get a specialized low-dose CT scan of your chest annually to look for any signs of the disease,

Radon may enter your house through cracks in the walls or flooring and cause a hazard. Radon levels are more significant in the Northeast, southern Appalachia, the Midwest, and the northern plains, but any residence might be impacted. Check out the Environmental Protection Agency's radon information page to determine whether you live in a high-radon zone and to learn how to test your home.

Colon and Rectal Cancer

Eight percent of all cancer diagnoses and eight percent of female cancer deaths are related to colon and rectal malignancies. A woman's likelihood of colon or rectal cancer is 1 in 24.

Although young people and teens can develop colon and rectal cancers, most instances are discovered in adults 50 years of age and older. The American Society for Clinical Oncology reports that the average age at which women are diagnosed with colon cancer is 72 (and the average age at diagnosis for males is 68). In addition to age, there are several other risk factors, some of which are under your control:

A history of colorectal cancer or polyps in oneself or one's family

Suffering from an inflammatory bowel condition, such as Crohn's disease or ulcerative colitis

Inactivity

Smoking

And excessive alcohol consumption

A diet deficient in fruits and vegetables and excessive in red or processed meat

Being overweight or obese

Type 2 diabetes

Being Ashkenazi (a Jew of Eastern European heritage) or African-American

Early diagnosis saves lives, particularly in the case of colon and rectal cancers. Since aberrant cells in the colon typically take 10 to 15 years to increase, getting frequent screening colonoscopies to check for polyps and remove them before they become abnormal might help you prevent some of the most severe side effects of these malignancies. According to current standards, you should undergo a colonoscopy at age 50, but it is advisable to discuss your condition with your doctor to see if you should get one sooner.

Additionally, several studies have demonstrated a correlation between a decreased risk of colorectal cancer and consuming adequate calcium through food or supplements.

Reducing risk can also be achieved by consuming more fiber and limiting red and processed meats. Food particles in processed meats are so small that they stay in the colon as the food moves through it." Moreover, you have greater exposure to carcinogens because they aren't moving through the bowels as quickly" if the food contains carcinogens. Conversely, fiber lowers your risk by swiftly moving feces through the colon.

Uterine Cancer

Four percent of female cancer deaths and 7% of all cancer cases were related to uterine cancer. The likelihood of uterine cancer in a woman is 1 in 36. Known by many names, including endometrial cancer, uterine cancer is defined as cancer of the endometrium, the lining of the uterus. It is more common than ovarian or cervical cancers to affect the female reproductive system. It is not one of the gynecological cancers brought on by HPV, in contrast to cervical cancer.

Hormonal changes, especially estrogen-related ones, greatly influence your risk for uterine cancer. Uterine cancer, like breast cancer, can be fed by estrogen. Several factors can alter hormone levels and raise the risk of uterine cancer. These include taking birth control pills, estrogen after menopause, having more menstrual cycles overall, having previously or currently taken tamoxifen for breast cancer, never getting pregnant, being obese, having specific ovarian tumors, and having polycystic ovarian syndrome.

CHAPTER THREE

Link between Diet and Cancer

Your grocery shop decisions affect more than simply what you eat for supper. The healthiest diet to prevent cancer may consist of as much as possible of foods produced in the ground.

The American Cancer Society predicts that 1.9 million new cancer cases will be detected in the United States in 2022. Although specific individuals possess an increased hereditary susceptibility to cancer, studies indicate that food and nutrition alone might save roughly 25% of cancer occurrences worldwide. Daily dietary decisions are critical in cancer prevention, as many malignancies might take ten years or more to manifest.

Diets mainly focused on plants include many fruits, vegetables, and legumes with little to no meat or other animal products. According to research studies, vegans, or those who abstain from any animal products, such as fish, dairy, or eggs, seem to have the lowest cancer risks of any diet. Vegetarians had the second-lowest percentage, or those who abstain from meat but may consume fish or animal-derived items like milk or eggs.

Plant-based diets provide benefits beyond just exquisite flavor. They are brimming with phytochemicals, chemical substances shielding the body from harm. Moreover, phytochemicals impede bodily functions that promote the development of cancer. In addition to being high in fiber, plant-based diets have been demonstrated to reduce the incidence of colorectal and breast cancer.

Plant chemicals

Phytochemicals are advantageous. They shield against harm, reduce inflammation, and sabotage bodily processes that promote cancer growth.

Here are two of the most beneficial phytochemicals:

Antioxidants

This kind of phytochemical guards against harm to the body. Damage to a cell's DNA results in cancer. It leads to the uncontrollable division of aberrant cells, which can penetrate and damage healthy human tissue. Radiation, infections, and exposure to other substances can potentially harm cells. Additionally, oxidants produced by the body's normal metabolism can potentially damage cells. Antioxidants shield and repair cells by counteracting these damaging processes. Dark chocolate, apples with peel, avocados, artichokes, red cabbage, tea, coffee, almonds, and grains are a few foods strong in antioxidants.

Carotenoids

Since they are fat-soluble substances, they must be absorbed in the presence of a fat source. Numerous fruits, cereals, oils, and vegetables, including carrots, sweet potatoes, squash, spinach, apricots, green peppers, and leafy greens, naturally contain carotenoids. Because of their intense pigmentation, seek natural foods in red, orange, yellow, and green. Carotenoids include things like lutein, lycopene, and beta-carotene. They may lower the risk of cataracts, macular degeneration, cancer, and heart disease.

Alpha and gamma carotene are provitamins that are abundant in plant-based diets. These vitamins can be transformed into vitamin A when consumed. This vitamin is necessary for immunity, cell division, growth, vision, and reproduction. Antioxidant properties are also present in vitamin A.

Plant-based diets contain nutrients and phytochemicals that reduce the risk of cancer and other diseases separately and in combination. Eating plant-based foods alone is less effective than eating them in conjunction with other foods. According to prostate cancer research, eating broccoli and tomatoes together was more successful than eating either vegetable to slow the formation of tumors. This illustrates the potency of nutrients when meals are combined.

Plant-based fiber

Natural fiber content is high in plant-based diets. This has been demonstrated to lower insulin levels and lower the risk of cancer. A research indicated a 25% lower risk of breast cancer in later life for young women who consumed the highest levels of fiber in their diets. According to another studies, consuming 10 grams of fiber each day may reduce the risk of colon cancer by 10%.

Fiber and other carbohydrates can be fermented by healthy bacteria in the digestive tract to create substances that have been shown to support healthy colon growth and lower inflammation. Certain phytochemicals are changed into more functional or active forms by these microorganisms.

Eat for variety and color.

A plant-based diet has many beautiful possibilities. Try novel foods like fruits or vegetables or inventive ways to prepare mainstays.

The cost of fresh fruits and vegetables may be a deciding factor when choosing a menu for a plant-based diet. Frozen fruits and veggies make excellent substitutes. They cost less and are flash-frozen to retain nutrients. There are other canned alternatives for those on a more restrictive budget. Be sure to look for options without added sugar or salt.

To feel full and get the needed fiber and phytochemicals, try to include at least these amounts of food in your diet:

1.5 to 2.5 cups of fruit each day

2.5 to 4 cups of vegetables each day

3 to 5 ounces of whole grains each day

1.5 cups of legumes each week

Five to seven ounces of protein a day. Excellent protein sources include eggs, dairy products, tofu, and legumes. Or choose lean meats and stay away from processed meats.

Fats, three to five portions daily. A serving is equivalent to one-sixth of an avocado, four walnut halves, or one teaspoon of oil.

Shifting to a plant-based diet

Consuming only plant-based foods doesn't have to be your only option. Making small, practical improvements is more feasible and sustainable for most individuals. Here are a few methods for doing this:

Start your day off right.

For a filling and nutritious breakfast that will give you the energy to take on the day, try whole-grain oats, buckwheat, or quinoa with fruit.

Experiment with meatless meals.

Accept "Meatless Mondays" and experiment with a different meatless meal each week.

Treat meat like a condiment.

Use just enough meat for flavor rather than as the main course.

Use legumes for bulk.

In some recipes, you may reduce the quantity of meat by adding more beans, lentils, or vegetables. You won't feel deprived because these meals take up more room on your plate.

Fill your plate with fruits and vegetables first.

For lunch and dinner, fill roughly half of your plate with fruits and vegetables.

Foods to Avoid

Your mental list of things to avoid is already in place if your therapy has resulted in adverse effects like nausea, taste changes, or mouth sores. Nonetheless, some foods—regardless of how delicious they may sound—are best avoided since they increase the risk of foodborne disease, sometimes known as food poisoning.

Food poisoning should not be taken lightly because specific treatments might impair your immune system for many weeks following their completion (longer if you had a stem cell or bone marrow transplant). A foodborne disease can have detrimental effects.

Eating raw or undercooked food is the most frequent way to get food poisoning. While germs are destroyed during proper cooking, they can still increase on prepared food if refrigerated or left out for an extended period. When food is handled by someone with a virus or other "bug" on them, it can also become contaminated.

It's crucial to follow food safety regulations and use additional caution when handling, preparing, and storing food.

Nonetheless, even if they may have eaten certain foods without any issues in the past, some people who are undergoing or have just ended cancer treatment should altogether avoid them. These consist of:

Cold hot dogs or deli lunch meat (cold cuts)—Always cook or reheat until the meat is steaming hot.

Raw, dry-cured salami

Raw milk and milk products that haven't been pasteurized, such as raw milk yogurt

Soft cheeses such as Brie, Camembert, feta, and goat cheese, queso fresco/Blanco, and blue-veined (a sort of blue cheese) created from unpasteurized milk

Smoked fish

Deli-prepared salads with egg, ham, chicken, or seafood

Refrigerated pâté—sorry foodies!

Unwashed fresh produce, particularly leafy greens that might conceal contaminants and dirt

Unpasteurized cider or fruit juice

Lucerne sprouts or other raw sprouts

Beef, particularly ground beef, or other raw or undercooked meat and poultry

Uncooked or raw shellfish, such as oysters, might harbor the hepatitis A virus. It is essential to boil these foods to eradicate the infection thoroughly.

Commercially frozen fish, especially those labeled "sushi-grade" or "sashimi-grade," is safer than other fish, but consult your physician, dietitian, or another member of your healthcare team before consuming sushi and sashimi, which frequently contain raw fish.

Undercooked eggs, such as soft boiled, over easy, and poached

Raw, unpasteurized eggs or foods made with raw egg, such as homemade raw cookie dough

How do plant-based foods fight cancer?

Plant-based diets and products can prevent cancer in several ways. Taking whole foods—rather than supplements—is the most effective approach to benefit from their anti-cancer properties. Generally, eating a nutritious diet is more important than knowing if a food is organic or adequately prepared.

Carotenoids

Carotenoids include beta-carotene (found in carrots), lutein (found in spinach), and lycopene (found in tomatoes) are sources of antioxidants. Antioxidants help protect your cells from damage that might lead to the development of malignant cells.

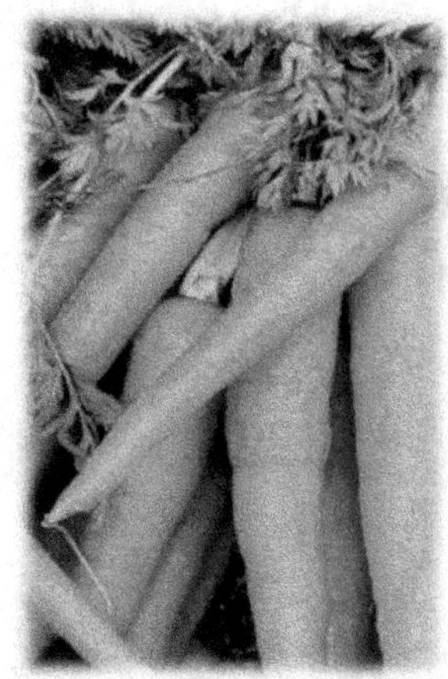

Greens

Leafy greens, which are high in folate, help create new DNA and occasionally fix damaged DNA. Your genetic abnormalities can cause malignant cells to grow from healthy ones.

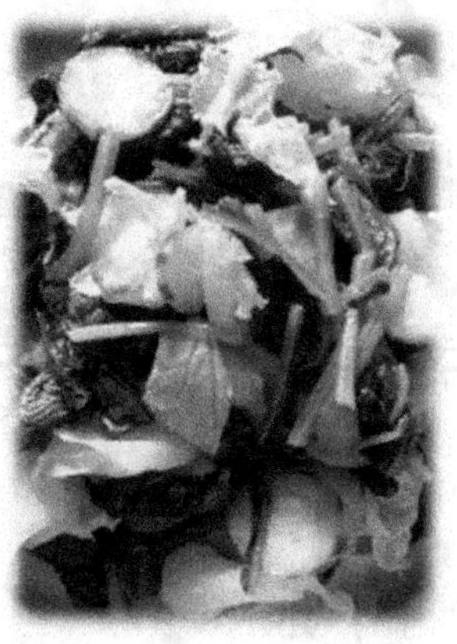

In the fight against cancer, cruciferous vegetables—those with flowers that resemble crosses—have several benefits.

They contain sulforaphane, which has the ability to prevent the initiation of several cancers. Furthermore, sulforaphane may stimulate the body's defense system against cancer by naturally killing cells.

Second, hormone-receptive cancers like breast cancer are successfully prevented and postponed by the indoles they contain.

Beans, Legumes and Soy ──────────────

Similar to cruciferous veggies, beans have several anti-cancer properties. Anti-cancer compounds found in beans include protease inhibitors, potentially reducing tumor development.

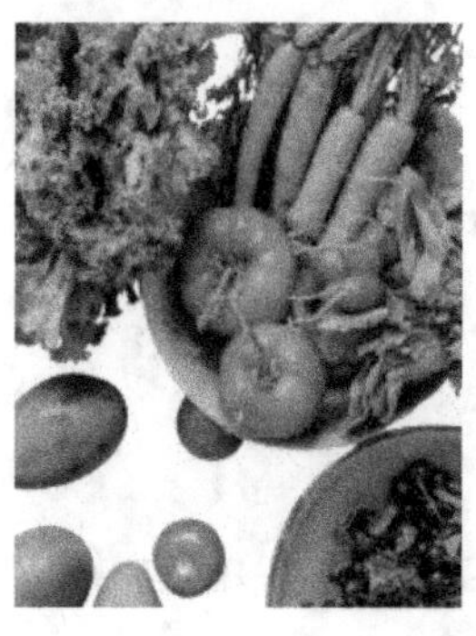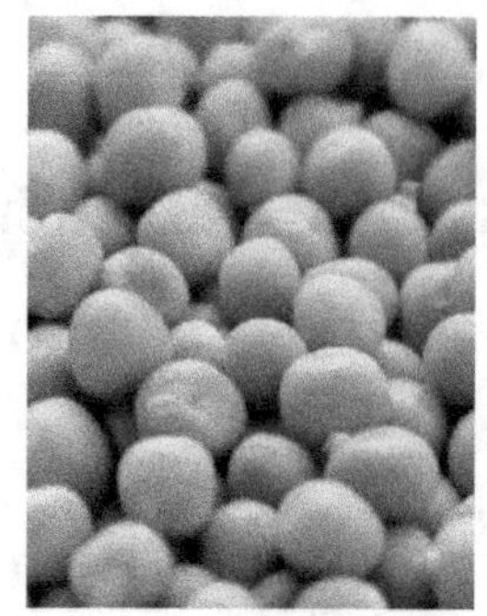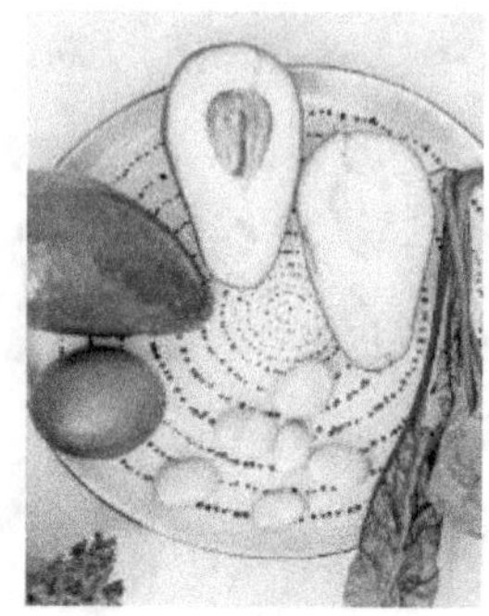

• Phytates, which have the potential to halt or prevent certain malignancies.

• Manganese, which aids in the formation of an enzyme that shields cells from harm.

• Quercetin and kaempferol, which have anti-inflammatory and antioxidant qualities.

Beans are best eaten cooked to prevent proteins called lectins from upsetting your stomach. These proteins are known as lectins. Although canned beans have fewer nutrients than fresh beans, you should still consume them because they don't contain BPA.

The easiest way to avoid GM plants is to consume organic soy. What you may have heard about soy's link to hormone-sensitive malignancies is untrue. Soy is safe for various diseases, according to a plethora of research conducted after 2009, including ones from the American Cancer Society.

Whole Grains, Oats, & More

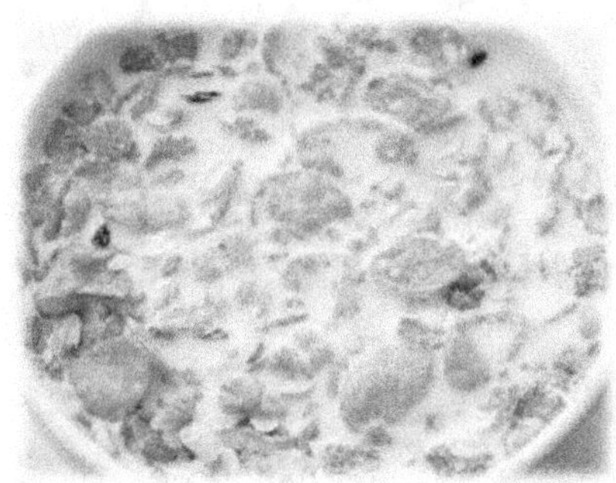 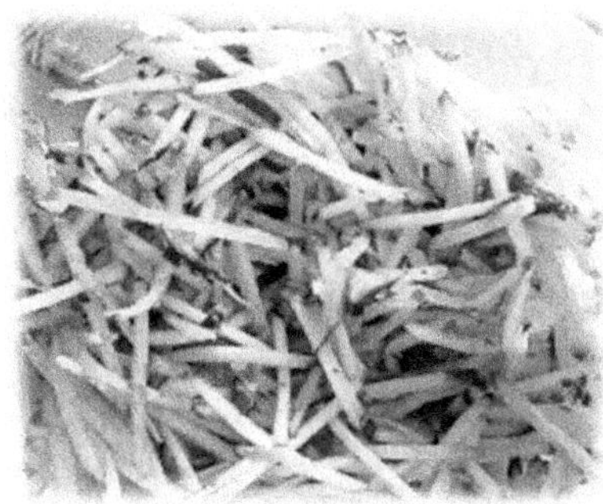

Low-glycemic carbohydrates such as whole grains and oats can be advantageous when taken in moderation. Low-glycemic foods avoid blood sugar spikes, which can make your body store more fat. Oats are a good source of manganese and B vitamins.

• *The mineral selenium enhances the immune system's capacity to fight cancer.*

• *Beta-glucan, which fortifies the immune system.*

47

• Plant lignans, which protect against hormone-sensitive cancers.

Seasonings

There are unexpectedly good benefits to seasoning food in terms of cancer prevention. Certain fresh or dried spices can reduce inflammation and provide antioxidants, two critical components of cancer prevention.

Turmeric spice has seven different methods to fight cancer. It becomes 1000% more soluble in your body when mixed with black pepper.

Crushed or chopped garlic is best when let sit for ten minutes before cooking.

Healthy Oils

Some oils can potentially prevent cancer and are far healthier than others. Consume these meals and prepare them using these oils.

• A lot of nuts are great providers of healthy fats and protein that can help decrease cholesterol.

• *Walnuts may lower the incidence and recurrence of breast cancer, according to recent research.*

• *For salad dressings and low-temperature cooking, use olive oil.*

Foods Having Additional Anti-Cancer Qualities

• *Berries include anthocyanins, which can inhibit the growth of cancer cells.*

In addition to tomatoes, watermelon is an excellent source of lycopene.

• *EGCG, present in white and green teas, can help stop tumors from attracting blood vessels to support their growth.*

The carefully chosen whole-food plant-based recipes that will act as your armor and a powerful ally against this terrible enemy known as cancer will be covered in the upcoming chapter. Go on to the next and let the path to recovery start.

CHAPTER FOUR

Breakfast Recipes

Scrambled Turmeric Tofu with Greens

Total time: 20 minutes   Number of Servings 6

Ingredients

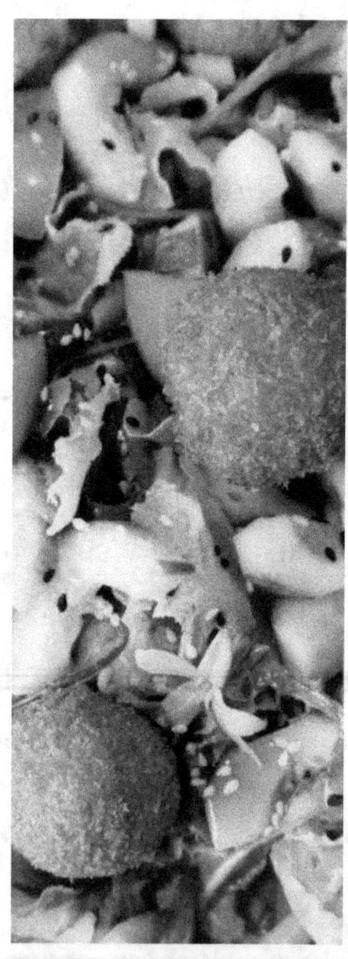

2 Tbsp. nutritional yeast

2 tsp. turmeric

1/4 tsp. smoked paprika

1/4 tsp. black pepper

Pinch sea salt (optional)

2 Tbsp. plain, unsweetened soymilk

1 Tbsp. extra-virgin olive oil

2 green onions, sliced

2 cloves garlic, minced

6 oz. (about 2 1/4 cups) sliced mushrooms

2 cups loosely packed chopped greens (e.g., mustard, collard, spinach, kale)

1/4 cup sun-dried tomatoes, chopped

1 14-oz. package of extra-firm tofu

Directions

- After taking the tofu out of the package, press it by wrapping it in paper towels, putting two plates on each other, and pressing for five minutes to let the excess liquid drip off.
- Transfer the tofu to a bowl and use your hands to crumble it into a crumbly consistency. Add the soymilk, nutritional yeast, smoked paprika, black pepper, and optional salt. Put away.
- For around five minutes, sauté green onions, garlic, and mushrooms in heated olive oil in a pan.
- Add the sun-dried tomatoes, chopped greens, and crumbled tofu. Sauté for approximately two minutes or until the greens begin to wilt.
- Serve immediately.

Nutritional Information:

Calories: 152

Total fat: 9 g

Cholesterol: 0 mg

Carbohydrates: 8 g

Protein: 14 g

Chickpea Crepes with Spinach and Mushroom Pesto

Total time: 70 minute   Number of Servings 6

Ingredients

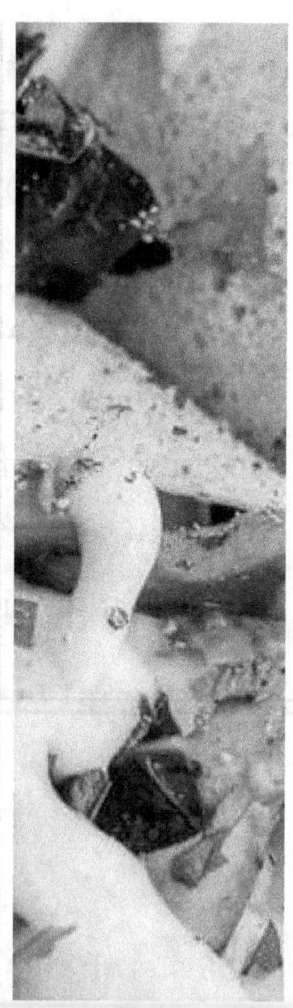

1/4 cup finely chopped red onion

1/3 cup finely chopped red bell pepper

6 oz. cremini mushrooms, thinly sliced (about 2 cups)

1 box (5 oz.) baby spinach

2 Tbsp. prepared pesto

Salt and freshly ground black pepper to taste

Crepes:

1 cup chickpea flour

2 Tbsp. extra-virgin olive oil

1 tsp. finely chopped fresh rosemary

1/4 tsp. salt

1 cup water

2 tsp. Soft buttery spread (if using skillet)

Directions

- In a medium bowl, whisk chickpea flour, oil, rosemary and salt with 1 cup water until mixture is smooth. Let batter sit 20-30 minutes to thicken. Before cooking, stir to loosen any clumps.

- For crepes, set a non-stick pan over medium-high heat until drops of water flicked into the pan ball up and bounce. With one hand, hold the pan up at a 45-degree angle. Pour ¼ cup batter near the top of the pan, rotating the pan as you pour so the batter flows into the 6-7-inch round crepe. Cook until crepe is golden on bottom, 1-2 minutes. Using a large spatula, flip and cook until the crepe is lightly golden on the bottom, about 30 seconds. Transfer the crepe to a large plate. Cover each crepe with wax paper.

- Suppose you are not filling the crepes immediately; let it cool to room temperature and cover the plate with plastic wrap. Hold crepes at room temperature for up to 8 hours and refrigerate for 24 hours.

- For filling, in a medium skillet, heat oil over medium-high heat. Add onion and cook, stirring for 2 minutes. Add red peppers and stir until onions are translucent for 5 minutes. Add mushrooms and cook, stirring occasionally, until the mixture looks wet, for another 5-6 minutes. Add spinach, stirring to wilt leaves. Cook, stirring often, until most of the moisture has evaporated and the filling is tender, for 8 minutes.

- If crepes have been made ahead, wrap them in foil and warm at 250 degrees F for 20 minutes. Mix pesto with 2 tbsp warm water to assemble crepes in a small bowl. Stir pesto into the filling. Arrange a crepe on a plate. Spoon ⅙ filling over the bottom half of each crepe, then gently fold the crepe in half over the filling. Repeat with remaining crepes and filling. If desired, garnish the plate with some mesclun leaves and strawberries. Serve immediately.

Nutritional Information:

170 calories: 170

Total fat: 10 g

Cholesterol: 0 mg

Carbohydrates: 13 g

Protein: 5 g

Oatmeal with Fresh Fruit

Total time: 15 minutes   Number of Servings 6

Ingredient

1/2 cup old-fashioned rolled oats

1 1/4 cups almond milk, divided*

1 tsp. ground flaxseed, or to taste

1/8 tsp. cinnamon

1/2 cup chopped pineapple

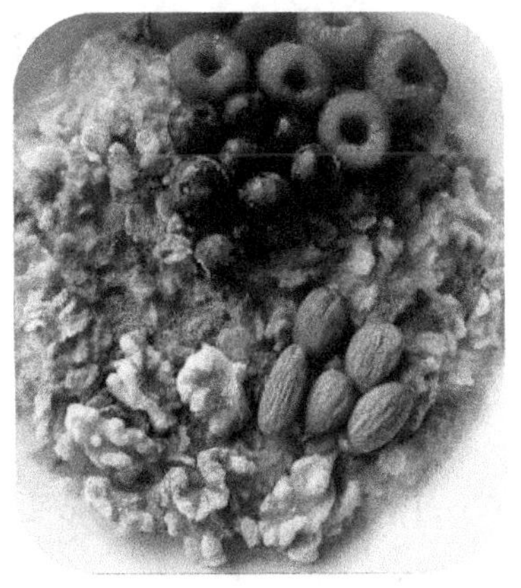

1/8 tsp. cinnamon

1/2 cup chopped pineapple

1/4 cup sliced strawberries

2 Tbsp. chopped walnuts, optional

1 tsp. honey, optional

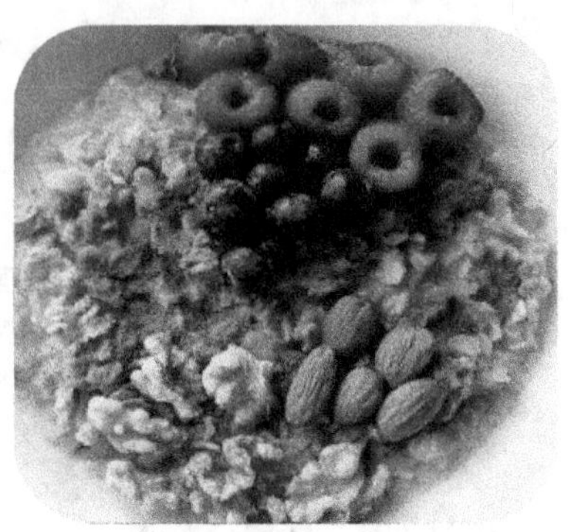

Directions

- Cook oats per package directions in a small pan with 1 cup of milk.

- Fill the serving dish with oats. Top oatmeal with ¼ cup warmed milk (if desired). Add some cinnamon and flaxseed.

- If preferred, garnish with honey, walnuts, pineapple, and strawberries.

Nutritional Information:

Calories: 370

Total fat: 16 g

Cholesterol: 0 mg

Carbohydrates: 50 g

Protein: 10 g

Herbed Spanish omelet

Total time: 60 minute   Number of Servings 2

Ingredients

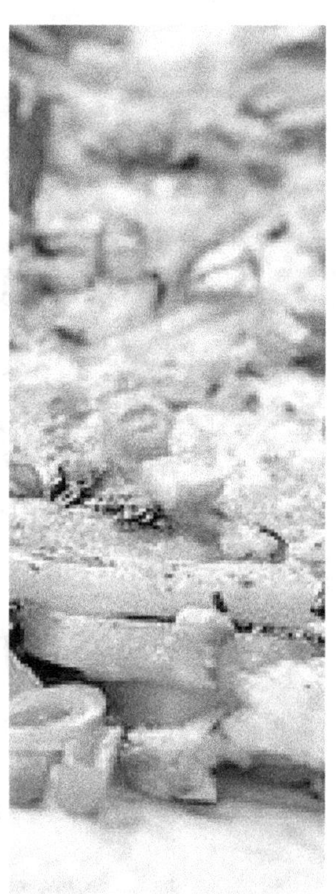

2 Tbsp. extra-virgin olive oil

1/2 cup diced red onion

2 cloves garlic, minced

1 lb. potatoes, peeled and diced

Or shredded

4 large whole eggs, lightly beaten

2 egg whites, lightly beaten

2 Tbsp. finely chopped fresh parsley

2 Tbsp. finely chopped fresh basil

And chives

Salt, to taste

Sprigs of fresh herbs to garnish

(Optional)

Directions

- Add the potatoes to a big pan. Pour water on top. Boil for three minutes, then remove the lid.

Take away from the flame. Potatoes should be soft but not mushy after about ten minutes of steaming covered. Make sure to drain well.

- Oil should be heated over medium heat in a deep 10-inch nonstick pan. Put garlic and onion in. Cook while stirring periodically for about 8 minutes. Cook for a further five minutes after adding the potatoes.

- Combine egg whites and whole eggs. Stir in chives, basil, and parsley. If preferred, season with salt. Over the potatoes in the heated skillet, pour the mixture. Once the omelette's bottom is brown, reduce heat and cook it uncovered for about ten minutes.

- Toast the top, if desired, in a toaster oven. Garnish with sprigs of fresh herb. Serve the dish right away.

Nutritional Information:

Calories: 240

Total fat: 12 g

Cholesterol: 185 mg

Carbohydrates: 23 g

Protein: 11 g

Apricot Pecan Bars

Total time: 40 minutes   Number of Servings

Ingredients

3 cups quick cooking oats

1/2 cup pecans, chopped

3 cups unsweetened grain cereal (cheerios or shredded wheat)

2 cups dried apricots, chopped

1/4 cup whole-wheat flour

12 oz. silken tofu, drained

1 large egg

1/2 cup applesauce

1/2 cup canola oil

3/4 cup honey

1/2 tsp. salt

1 Tbsp. lemon zest, freshly grated

1 Tbsp. vanilla extract

Canola oil cooking spray

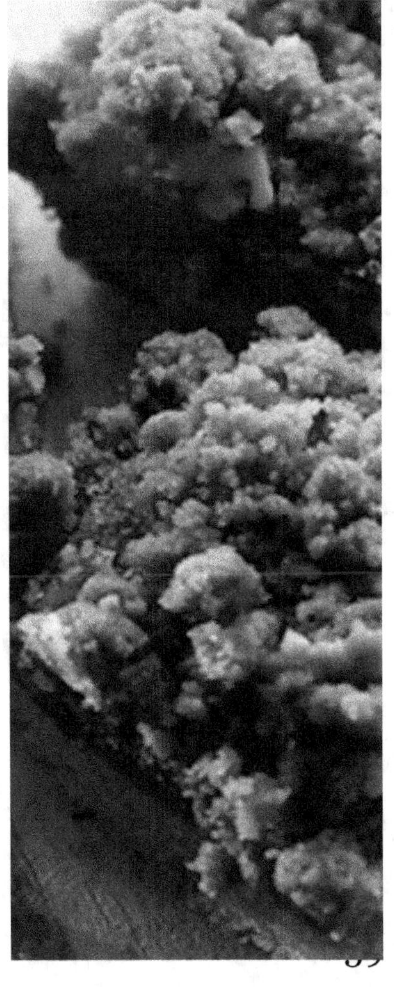

Directional:

- Set oven temperature to 350°F.

- Line a large (15 x 10 inch) baking dish with oats and pecans. Bake for 8 to 10 minutes or until aromatic and gently browned.

- Transfer to a sizable mixing basin, then whisk the flour, cereal, and apricots.

- In a blender, puree the tofu, egg, applesauce, oil, honey, vanilla, and zest of one lemon until smooth. Create a well in the middle of the mixture of oats and tofu, then fold in until thoroughly incorporated. Apply cooking spray to a 9x13 baking dish and evenly distribute the ingredients.

- Bake for 35 to 40 minutes or until golden brown and firm to the touch in the center. Allow it to cool fully in the dish, then use a sharp knife to cut into bars.

Nutritional Information:

Calories: 190

Total fat: 8 g

Cholesterol: 10 mg

Carbohydrates: 30 g

Protein: 4 g

Pumpkin Spice Overnight Oats

Total time: 5 minutes (plus overnight soaking)   Number of Servings 2

Ingredients

1/2 cup of almond milk, unsweetened (or any milk)

1/2 cup rolled Oats

1/3 cup plain, low-fat Greek yoghurt

1 teaspoon of ground flaxseed

2 tablespoons pureed pumpkin

1 teaspoon of maple syrup

1/2 teaspoon vanilla extract

1/2 tsp of cinnamon powder

1/4 tsp. of ginger powder

1/4 tsp. nutmeg powder

A pinch of salt

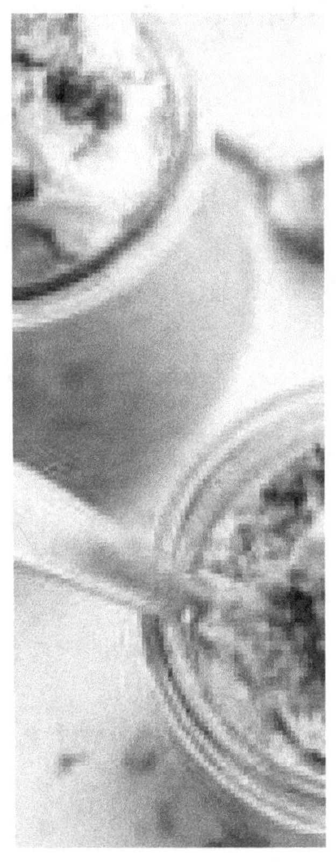

Directional:

- Combine all ingredients in a medium-sized mixing bowl and stir to combine.
- Fill a mason jar with a tight-fitting lid.
- Store overnight in the refrigerator.

Nutritional Information:

Calories: 340

Total fat: 7 g

Cholesterol: 10 mg

Carbohydrates: 52 g

Protein: 16 g

Sautéed Chard with Feta and Egg Breakfast Toast

Total time: 15 minutes   Number of Servings

Ingredients:

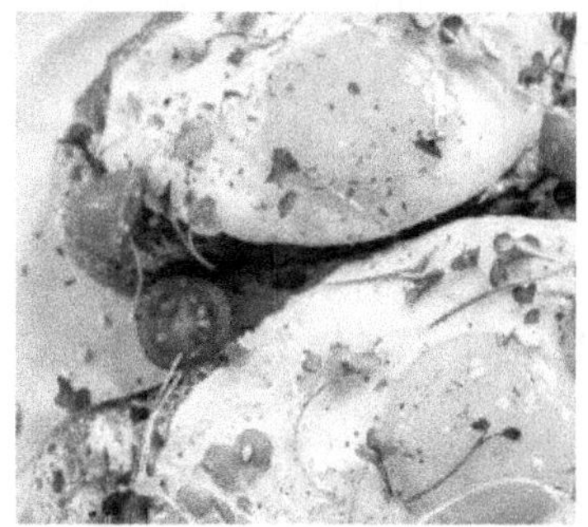

Directions:

- Toast bread.
- Chard is sautéed in olive oil until it becomes tender and has shrunk by roughly half.
- Spread it over your bread, then top with a hard-boiled egg, feta, and more.

Notes:

- *You may use spinach or kale in place of chard.*
- *While sautéing the chard, you can choose to add a squeeze of lemon, minced garlic, or crushed red pepper flakes.*
- *Hard-boiled egg, sliced thinly.*

Nutritional Information:

Calories: 340

Total fat: 12 g

Cholesterol: 190 mg

Carbohydrates: 15 g

Protein: 7 g

Cottage Cheese, Cucumber and Tomato

Total time: 10 minutes   Number of Servings 2

Ingredients:

1 slice whole grain bread

¼ cup reduced-fat cottage cheese

4-5 thin cucumber slices

2-3 thin tomato slices, cut into quarters

Cracked black pepper (to taste)

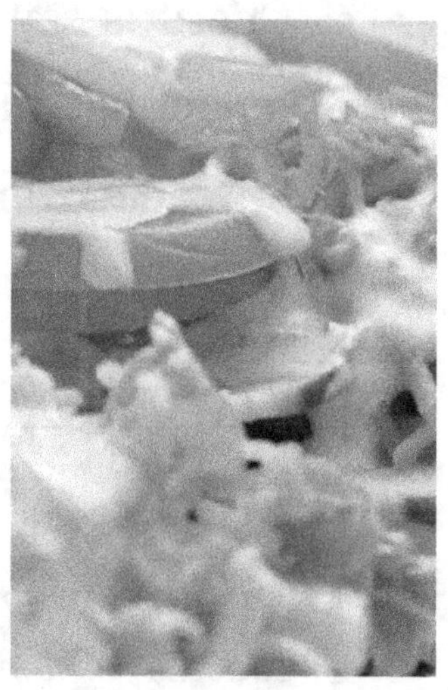

Directions

- Toast bread.

- On toast, spread cottage cheese.

- Add slices of tomato, cucumber, and black pepper on top.

Nutritional Information:

Calories: 150

Total fat: 3 g

Cholesterol: 5 mg

Carbohydrates: 19 g

Protein: 10 g

Peanut Butter Toast with Banana and Chia Seeds

Total time: 5 minutes   Number of Servings 2

Ingredients:

1 tsp. chia seed (or flaxseed)

1/2 banana, sliced

1 Tbsp. peanut butter

1 slice whole grain bread

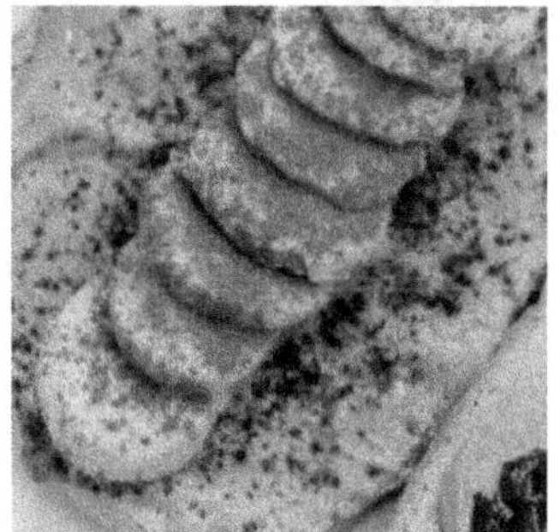

Directions:

- Toast bread.

- Toast with peanut butter on it.
- Add sliced banana and chia seeds on top.

Notes:

You may use flaxseed for chia seeds and almond butter for peanut butter.

Nutritional Information:

Calories: 150

Total fat: 11 g

Cholesterol: 0 mg

Carbohydrates: 34 g

Protein: 9 g

Mashed Avocado Toast with Feta and Pepitas Seeds Toast

Total time: 10 minutes   Number of Servings 2

Ingredients:

1 lemon wedge

1/3 avocado, mashed

1 tsp. feta cheese

1 tsp. pepitas (pumpkin seeds)

1 slice whole grain bread

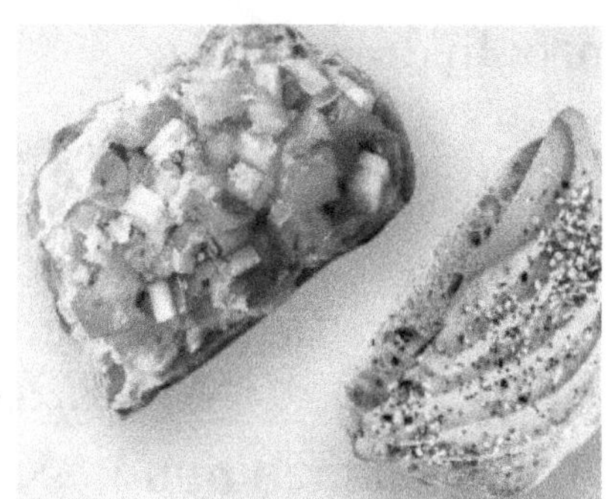

Directions

- Toast bread.
- Mash avocado and thoroughly combine it with lemon juice.
- Place everything on top of the bread.

Notes

Pomegranate seeds may be used instead of pumpkin seeds to give avocado toast some crunch and a lovely splash of color.

Nutritional Information:

Calories: 210

Total fat: 12 g

Cholesterol: 5 mg

Carbohydrates: 22 g

Protein: 6 g

Refried Beans, Pico and Sunny Side Egg Breakfast Toast

Total time: 20 minutes   Number of Servings 2

Ingredient

1 sunny side up egg

*2 Tbsp. refried beans, low sodium**

1 Tbsp. Pico de Gallo

1 slice whole grain bread

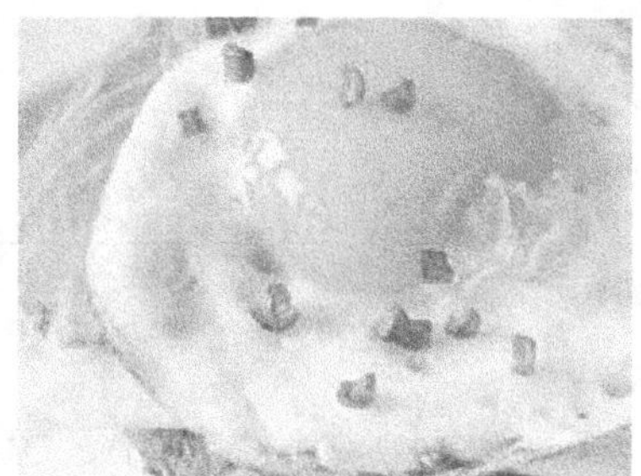

Directions

- Toast bread.
- Use a burner or microwave to reheat the beans.
- Cook egg sunny-side up.
- Place everything on top of the bread.

Notes:

* Fresh pinto or black beans can also be used.

Nutritional Information:

Calories: 190

Total fat: 7 g

Cholesterol: 185 mg

Carbohydrates: 19 g

Protein: 11 g

Bagel Avocado Toast with Salmon

Total time: 15 minutes   Number of Servings 2

Ingredients

4 (4 ounces each) wild Alaska salmon fillets, preferably cut from the thinner tail end

2 Tbsp. olive oil

1 egg white

2 Tbsp. cornstarch

3 Tbsp. sesame seeds

3 Tbsp. poppy seeds

1 Tbsp. dried minced onion

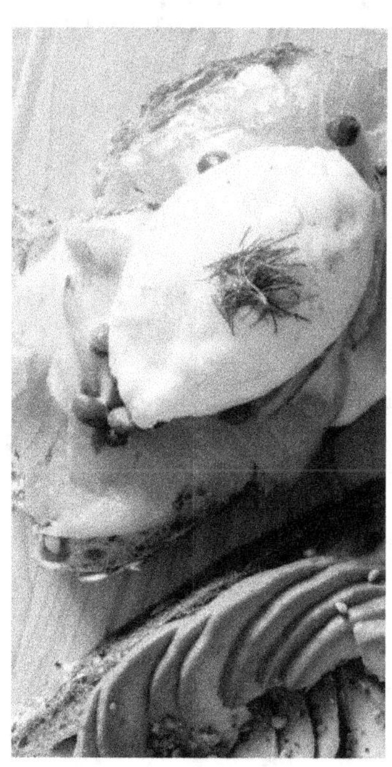

2 tsp. dried minced garlic

1/2 tsp. coarse or flaked salt

2 whole grain bagels, halved and toasted

1 avocado, seeded, sliced, and scooped

2 small lemons, quartered

Salt and pepper, to taste

8 slices tomato (4 if tomatoes are large)

4 slices red onion

4 tsp. capers (optional)

1 tsp. chopped parsley, for garnish

Directions

- Combine the sesame seeds, poppy seeds, salt, dried onion, and dried garlic in a basin.

- Using a fork, blend the egg white and cornstarch in a small bowl until smooth. Apply the egg-white mixture to the salmon fillets' skinless sides. Arrange the seeds onto a dish. Coat the salmon fillets by pressing their skinless side into the seeds.

- Heat the oil in a large nonstick frying pan over medium heat. Cook the salmon for one to two minutes, or until golden brown, with the seed side down. Check the seeds after one minute since they brown rapidly. After 2 to 3 minutes, flip the salmon over and continue cooking it for another 2 to 3 minutes or until the internal temperature of the thickest section of the fish reaches 125° F. The precise time will change based on how thick the fillets are.

- While you make the bagels, transfer the cooked salmon to a platter and loosely cover it with foil. While it rests, the salmon will continue to cook.

- Toast the bagel halves and put them out on a chopping board. Place the avocado slices on top. Use a fork to mash them, or leave them in slices. Add a little of pepper, salt, and lemon juice. Top each half of a bagel with two slices of tomato.

- Top each bagel with a slice of grilled salmon. Serve with the remaining lemon wedges on top, garnished with onion slices, capers, and parsley.

Nutritional Information:

Calories: 190

Total fat: 7 g

Cholesterol: 185 mg

Carbohydrates: 19 g

Protein: 11 g

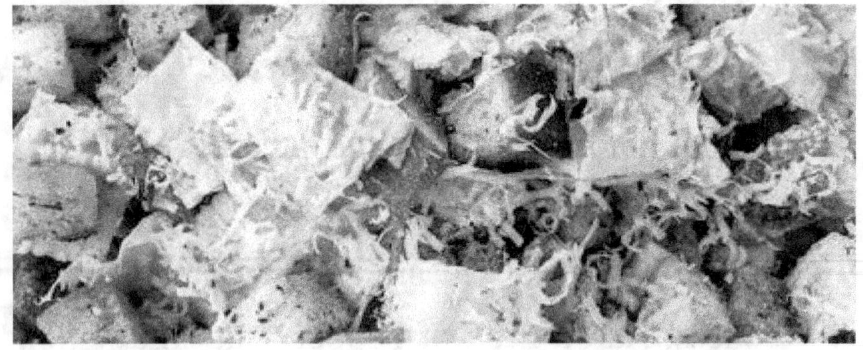

CHAPTER FIVE

LUNCH RECIPES

Lentil Walnut Tacos with Cabbage Lime Slaw

Total time: 35 minutes   Number of Servings 2

Ingredients

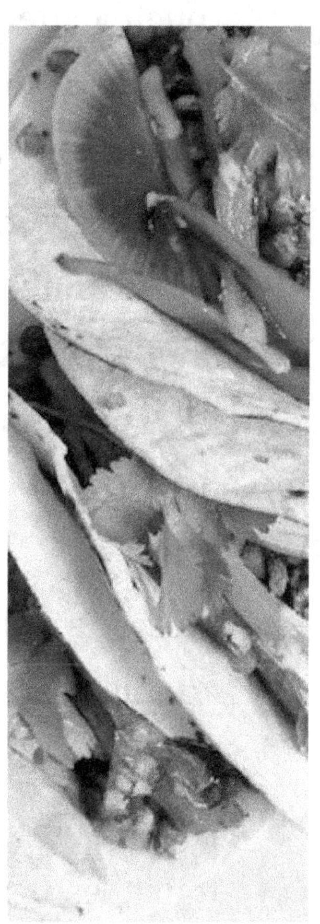

3 cups water*

1 1/2 cups crimson lentils

1 cup walnuts

1 tablespoon tamari**

2 garlic cloves, peeled

1/2 cup sun-dried tomatoes

1/2 teaspoon cumin powder

1 teaspoon chili powder

1 teaspoon apple cider vinegar**

3 cups shredded red cabbage

2 green onions1/2 cup cilantro

2 tablespoons olive oil*

1 lime

2 teaspoons agave syrup

12 corn taco shells

1/2 teaspoon crushed red pepper flakes

**sauce mix

Directions:

- After rinsing, dry the fruit. Cut the sun-dried tomatoes and green onions coarsely, and remove the bulbs. Chop the cilantro leaves roughly after removing them from their stems and discarding them. Chop up the garlic. Halve the lime and set it aside.

- Bring three cups of water to a boil for the lentils in a medium pot. Reduce the heat to a simmer after adding the lentils. Cook lentils uncovered for approximately 25 minutes or until they are tender. After removing any extra water, keep it aside.

- Pulse the walnuts in a food processor until they are finely crushed to produce the lentil walnut crumble. Pulse two or three more times to thoroughly mix the tamari, garlic, sun-dried tomatoes, cumin, chili powder spice combination, and apple cider vinegar.

- When the mixture is well combined and crumbly, add the cooked lentils and pulse again, adding a few tablespoons of water as necessary. Set the crumble aside.

- Mix the cabbage, chopped green onions, crushed red pepper, and cilantro in a large mixing basin to form the cabbage slaw. Pour the agave syrup and two tablespoons of olive oil into a bowl, add the slaw, and squeeze in the lime juice. Blend well.

- There should be enough crumble filling to make 8–12 tacos. To assemble the tacos, divide them evenly among the taco shells. Place a generous amount of the cabbage slaw on top, and enjoy!

Nutritional Information:

Calories: 660

Fat: 29g

Carbohydrates: 79g

Protein: 28g

Mango and Black Bean Salad

Total time: 11 minutes   Number of Servings 4

Ingredients:

2 large mangoes, peeled and chopped

1 red bell pepper, seeded and diced

½ of a red onion, finely diced

1 jalapeno, seeds, and ribs removed, then minced

1 can of black beans, drained and rinsed

1 ½ cups corn kernels

¼ cup chopped cilantro leaves

2 tablespoons olive oil

1 tablespoon lime juice

Salt and pepper to taste

½ teaspoon ground cumin

½ teaspoon chili powder

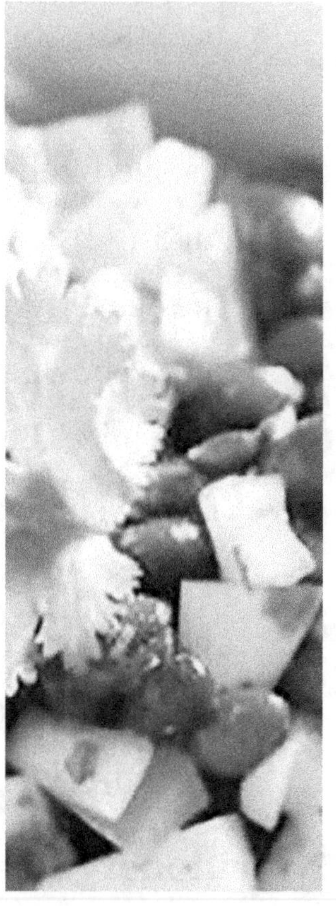

Directions:

- Combine bell pepper, onion, jalapeño, black beans, mango, corn, and cilantro in a big bowl.

- Mix the olive oil, lime juice, chili powder, cumin, and salt and pepper in a small bowl.
- After adding the dressing to the vegetable mixture, gently stir everything until well combined. Serve.

Nutritional Information:

Calories: 178kcal

Carbohydrates: 27g

Protein: 2g

Fat: 8g

Zucchini Noodles with Pesto and Tomatoes

Total time: 25 minutes   Number of Servings 4

Ingredients:

2 cups packed fresh basil leaves

2 cloves garlic

1/3 cup extra-virgin olive oil

2 teaspoons fresh lemon juice

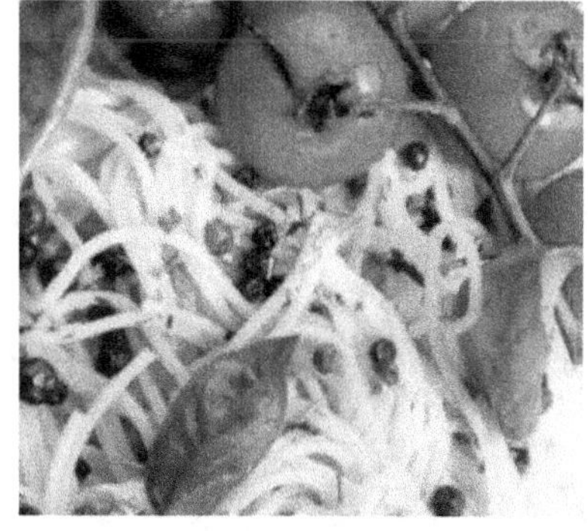

Directions:

- Use a mandoline or julienne peeler to cut the zucchini into thin noodles. Put away. In a food processor, combine the garlic and basil and pulse until finely chopped. Slowly add the olive oil in a steady stream with the food processor running.

- With a rubber spatula, stop the machine and scrape down the food processor's sides. Incorporate the Parmesan cheese and lemon juice. Pulse to combine. Add pepper and salt for seasoning.

- Add the pesto to the zucchini noodles and mix. Toss until noodles made of zucchini are evenly coated. Add tomatoes on top if using. Serve cold or at room temperature.

Note: You are welcome to boil the zucchini noodles if you like. Toss in the zucchini pesto noodles and cook over medium heat in a skillet. It takes a few minutes at most.

Nutritional Information:

Calories: 224kcal

Carbohydrates: 7g

Protein: 5g

Fat: 20g

Easy vegan spinach & artichoke quiche

Total time: 2 hrs. 15 min   Number of Servings 8

Ingredients

Crust (or use a store-bought crust)
1 1/4 cups all-purpose flour
1/2 teaspoon salt
*4–5 tablespoons ice water**
*1/2 cup solid coconut oil**
2 cloves garlic, finely minced (optional but recommended)

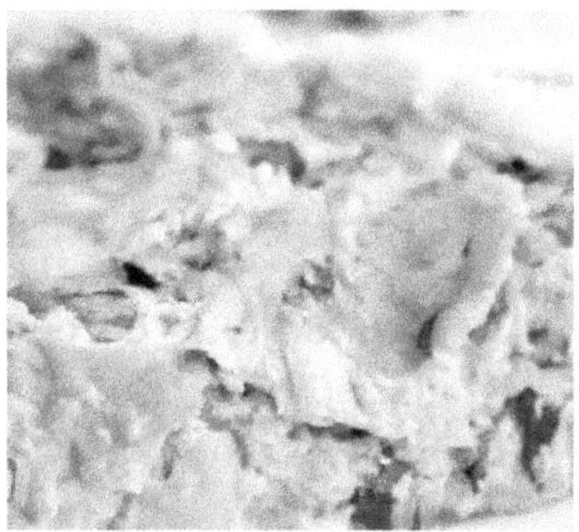

FILLING

1 (14 oz.) package extra-firm tofu, drained

3/4 teaspoon salt, plus more to taste

1 tablespoon lemon juice

2 tablespoons nutritional yeast flakes

1–3 tablespoons almond milk, as needed

1/4 teaspoon turmeric

1/4 teaspoon Kala namak (Indian black salt), to taste (optional, for eggy flavor)

2 tablespoons chopped fresh herbs (we used parsley)

1/3 cup vegetable broth

1/2 medium onion, finely diced

2 garlic cloves, finely minced

2 cups packed baby spinach, roughly chopped

6 oz. Marinated artichoke hearts, drained and roughly chopped, patted dry with paper towels.

Other optional vegetables

1 medium leek, finely chopped (white and light green parts only)

1 cup mushrooms, finely chopped

1/2 bell pepper, finely diced

Directions:

CRUST

- Combine the all-purpose flour, salt, and minced garlic in a large basin and stir until well combined. Using a fork or party cutter, gradually cut in the coconut oil until the mixture is the consistency of sand. Two teaspoons of cold water should be added until the dough is wet enough to form a ball. In total, we used eight tablespoons.

- Form the dough into a disk, cover it with plastic wrap*, and refrigerate to firm for at least half an hour.

- After the dough solidifies, take out a pie pan. Don't grease the pan. Make careful to produce a crust by pressing the dough evenly into the sides and bottom of the pie pan. You can add a crust pattern or crimp the edges if you'd like. Put the crust back in the fridge for half an hour.

- Set oven temperature to 375°F. Take the crust out of the fridge. Pie weights or dry beans can be added to the crust by placing a large piece of parchment paper on top. It will prevent it from collapsing. Put the crust in the oven and bake it mindlessly for fifteen minutes or until it is slightly brown around the edges.

- Remove the parchment paper and pie weights after taking the crust out of the oven. Make punctures in the crust's sides and bottom with a fork. Put the crust back in the oven for a further ten minutes, uncovered. Take out and place aside.

FILLING AND VEGETABLES

- Add two tablespoons of vegetable broth to a medium skillet set over medium heat. Add the leek, garlic, and onions once heated through.
- The garlic should be aromatic, and the onions should be transparent after 3–4 minutes of sautéing. Add more vegetable broth, one tablespoon at a time, to keep it from burning.
- When cooked, include the bell pepper and mushrooms. Simmer for a further 4 minutes or until tender.
- When every veggie has finished cooking, add the spinach to the saucepan after turning off the heat. After stirring the spinach well, cover

the saucepan and let it steam for five minutes. Add the artichokes and set aside.

- Add the tofu, turmeric, lemon juice, nutritional yeast, and black salt to a food processor. Mix until homogeneous. Add one tablespoon of almond milk to the mixture if it's crumbly until smooth.

- To taste, add salt. When the parsley is well incorporated but not entirely broken down, add it and pulse. Transfer to a large bowl. The cooked vegetable combination should be added and thoroughly mixed.

ASSEMBLY

- Spread the quiche mixture evenly in the pie shell after transferring it with a spatula. After placing the quiche in the oven, bake it for 25 to 30 minutes or until the top has deepened in color and the crust is golden.

- Take it out of the oven and let it be entirely cool before serving. It is preferable to refrigerate this quiche and serve it the following day. Have fun!

Nutritional Information:

Calories: 224kcal

Carbohydrates: 7g

Protein: 5g

Fat: 20g

Creamy Cauliflower and Chickpea Curry

Total time: 25 minutes   Number of Servings 4

Ingredient

1 red onion

4 garlic cloves

Inch of ginger

1 tbsp curry powder, medium

1 tsp ground cumin

1/2 tsp garam masala

1/4 tsp ground turmeric

1/4 tsp chilli powder

1/4 tsp salt

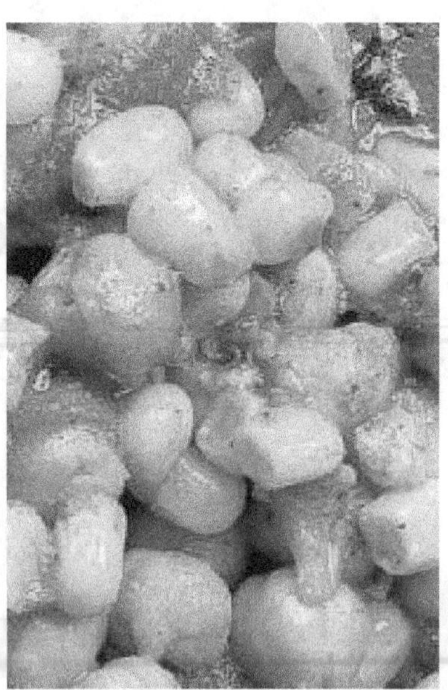

1 tin/400g tinned chopped tomatoes

1 tbsp tomato puree

1 tin/400ml full-fat coconut milk

1/2 cup/120ml vegetable stock

1 medium cauliflower (around 4 cups)

1 tin/400g chickpeas, drained

Optional toppings

Drizzle of vegan cream

Fresh coriander

Directions

- Warm up a tablespoon of oil in a big pan over medium heat.

- After a few minutes, add the finely chopped onion and continue to simmer. Next, include the grated ginger and chopped garlic.

- Stirring often to prevent burning, cook for one minute.

- Add the salt, turmeric, chili powder, garam masala, cumin, and curry powder. Simmer for about 30 seconds or until aromatic. If it's too dry, add a bit of extra oil.

- Add the tomato puree and diced tomatoes. Cook for a few minutes while stirring.

- Once smooth, transfer to a bowl, puree with a hand blender or in a blender, and then put back in the pan.

- Add the cauliflower, stock, and coconut milk. Bite-sized chunks of cauliflower should be cut; they shouldn't be too big or too little.

- After 10 to 15 minutes of simmering, add the chickpeas and cook for an additional five minutes.

- Although mushy, the cauliflower should still have some bite to it. Cook it for a little longer if you want it tender.

- Add some fresh coriander and coconut milk or vegan cream as garnish!

- Notes

- Will store it for two to three days in the refrigerator in an airtight container; to freeze this, I suggest freezing the sauce alone and then reheating it once the cauliflower and chickpeas have been added.

Nutritional Information:

Calories: 596

Carbohydrates: 57g

Protein: 20g

Fat: 36g

Spicy chickpea wraps with spinach and avocado

Total time: 10 minutes   Number of Servings 6

Ingredients

Large tortillas
Spinach
1/2 avocado per wrap
2 14 oz or 1 28 oz can of chickpeas, drained and rinsed (approx. 3.5 cups)
2–3 tbsp Sriracha sauce (start with 2 tbsp; add more as needed or to taste)
2–3 tbsp vegan mayo or tahini (start with 2 tbsp, add more as needed or to taste)
1–2 tbsp fresh lemon juice (start with 1 tbsp; add more as needed or to taste)

1 tsp garlic powder
Salt and pepper, to taste
1 cup lightly packed cilantro, chopped

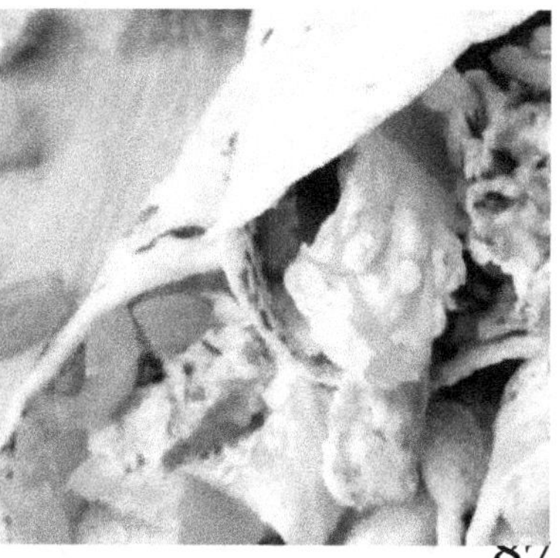

Directions

- The chickpeas can be mashed with a fork or potato masher in a bowl or placed in a food processor or blender and pulsed until they are mostly broken down. Though bulky, it should be beginning to come together.

- In a mixing dish, combine the chickpea mixture with all the ingredients except the avocado and spinach. Blend well. It should have the consistency of tuna salad or egg. Adjust the amount of mayo, lemon, and sriracha to get the right texture or taste.

- To create the wraps, fill each with a scoop of the chickpea mixture, then add avocado and spinach. If preferred, add salt and pepper for seasoning.

- Roll them up and enjoy!

Nutritional Information:

Calories: 130
Carbohydrates: 17 g
Protein: 6g
Fat: 5g

Lentil and Vegetable Stir-Fry avocado

Total time: 30 minutes   Number of Servings 4

Ingredients:

Stir Fry

2 tablespoons vegetable oil

¾ cup onion, sliced or diced

2-3 cloves garlic, minced

1 tablespoon ginger, chopped or finely grated

1 ½ cups bell pepper, sliced or diced (about 1 medium pepper)

¾ cup celery, sliced

¾ cup carrots, sliced

¾ cup zucchini, sliced

2 cups lentils, drained and rinsed (about 19oz canned)

½ cup cashews

Sauce

*4 tablespoons soy sauce, low sodium**

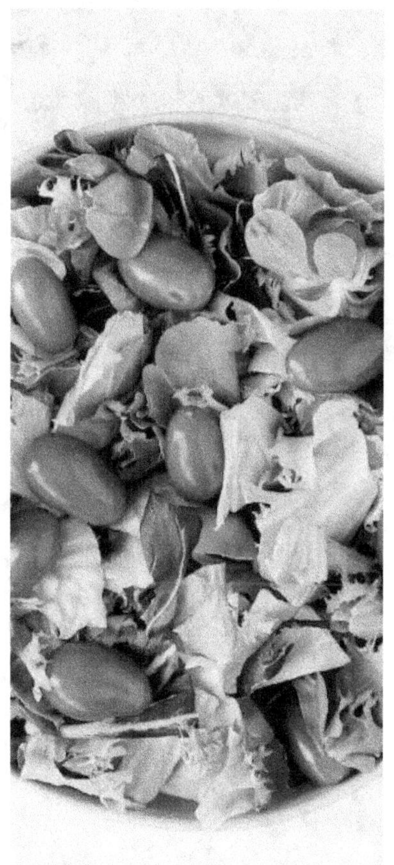

3 tablespoons hoisin sauce

2 tablespoons rice vinegar

2 tablespoons mirin **

½ tablespoon lime zest (about 1 lime)

2 tablespoons lime juice (about 1 lime)

1 tablespoon sesame oil

2 teaspoons brown sugar

2 teaspoons corn starch

To Serve

Green onion, sliced

White sesame seeds (or black sesame seeds)

Rice (or rice noodles)

Cashews (extra)

Directions

- As rice might take some time to cook if you plan to serve this stir fry with rice, start that process immediately. Rice noodles may be made at any time and cooked fast when served.

- Wash and chop all of the veggies before you start. I slice all the vegetables for this dish, but you may cut them as you wish.

- 1 ½ cups bell pepper, 2–3 cloves garlic, 1 tablespoon ginger, 1 cup onion, 1 cup celery, 1 cup carrots, and 1 cup zucchini

- Rinse and drain lentils from a can. If you'd like, you may also use freshly cooked lentils. For this dish, any lentil will work. However, brown or green are the best.

- Combine all the sauce ingredients in a dish or jar and whisk to combine well (or shake a jar with a cover). Set aside.

- Four tablespoons of soy sauce, three tablespoons of hoisin sauce, two tablespoons each of rice vinegar and mirin, half a tablespoon of lime zest and juice, one tablespoon of sesame oil, two teaspoons each of brown sugar and corn starch.

- In a big pan, preheat some vegetable oil over medium-high heat.

- Add the onion and stir-fry for one to two minutes or until it softens and becomes translucent.

- Add the carrots, celery, ginger, and garlic after that. Cook for about 2 minutes, stirring the ingredients often.

- After that, add the bell pepper and zucchini and simmer for two to three minutes or until the veggies are almost done (if you prefer softer vegetables, this might take longer).

- Add the lentils, cashews, and sauce to the pan when the veggies are almost done. Cook for an additional minute or two or until the sauce thickens. Once the sauce is in the pan, stir it often.

Serve

- Serve this stir fry over cooked rice noodles or over a side dish of rice. Serve with quinoa or another grain if you'd like. If you'd prefer something with fewer carbohydrates, cauliflower rice can also work.

- Add more cashews, sliced green onions, black or white sesame seeds, or any other desired garnish on top.

NOTES: * For a gluten-free alternative, use soy sauce instead of tamari. **You may also use it instead of cooking sherry or white wine.

Nutritional Information:

Calories: 424 kcal

Carbohydrates: 51 g

Protein: 16 g

Fat: 19 g

Spinach, mushroom & pepper stuffed shells

Total time: 30 minutes   Number of Servings 44

Ingredients

Salt & water for boiling pasta

1 (12-ounce) box jumbo shells pasta

2 cups mozzarella shredded & divided

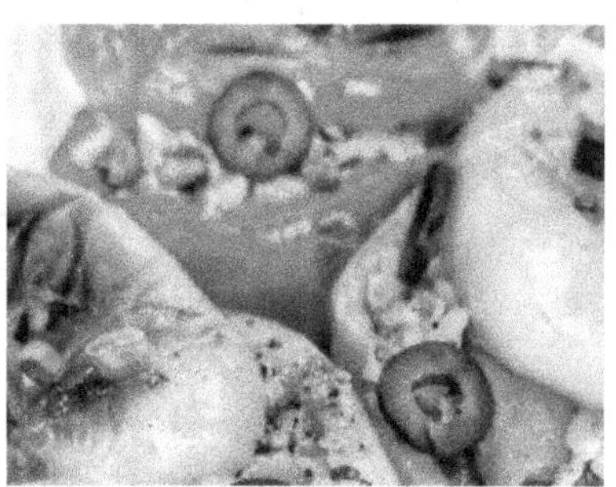

2 (24-ounce) jars of marinara sauce (or homemade)

1 egg

1/2 cup Parmesan cheese grated

1 (30-ounce) container of ricotta cheese (I use whole milk)

1 (12-ounce) jar of roasted red peppers, drained & chopped

1/8 teaspoon red pepper flakes (optional)

1/4 teaspoon pepper

1/2 teaspoon salt

1 teaspoon Italian seasoning

1 teaspoon garlic, minced

8 ounces sliced crimini (baby bella) mushrooms, chopped

1/2 sweet onion, chopped

1 tablespoon olive oil

2 (10-ounce) boxes of frozen chopped spinach, thawed & squeezed dry

Directions

- Set the oven's temperature to 375.

- Six quarts of boiling salted water (about three to four teaspoons of kosher salt) are needed.

- Fill a big skillet with oil and heat it to medium.

- Add red pepper flakes, onion, mushrooms, garlic, and Italian seasoning to the pan.

- Cook for approximately 8 minutes, stirring regularly, or until softened.

- Stir the spinach and peppers together until thoroughly mixed. Cut the heat and give it a little time to cool.

- Cook for approximately nine minutes (slightly less than the packaging says). The oven will cook them more.

- After draining, transfer the pasta to a baking sheet with an oiled rim. It will be able to cool slightly and separate as a result.

- Ricotta, Parmesan, egg, and one cup of mozzarella should all be combined in a big basin (or well mixed in a stand mixer). Toss to blend. Add the spinach mixture and stir.

- Fill the bottom of a 13" x 9" x 2" baking dish with roughly 1 1/2 cups of marinara sauce; distribute evenly.

- Place two to three teaspoons of filling into each shell. Put them in a pan. (I prefer to arrange them into a single layer of around 34 shells, then place them on a different little plate to bake or freeze separately.)

- After adding another 1 1/2 cups of sauce to the filled shells, top with the last cup of cheese.
- Wrap the dish with foil. Bake for 40 to 45 minutes with a lid on. After removing the foil, heat 10 to 15 minutes or until the cheese has melted.
- If preferred, serve with more heated marinara sauce on the side.

Nutritional Information:

Calories: 424 kcal

Carbohydrates: 51 g

Protein: 16 g

Fat: 19 g

Easy Sweet Potato and Black Bean Burrito Bowls

Total time: 45 minutes   Number of Servings 4

Ingredients:

Extra virgin olive oil

Kosher salt

1 tablespoon plus 1/2 tsp chili powder, divided

4 small sweet potatoes (about 2 lbs), chopped into 1-inch pieces

2 cups short-grain white or brown rice

2 limes, zest of one and juice of two, divided (about 2 tsp zest and ¼ cup juice)

1 cup fresh cilantro leaves and tender stems, finely chopped

2 avocados, diced

½ cup sour cream

Hot sauce, to taste

1 (15-oz) can of black beans, drained and rinsed

2 bell peppers, chopped

Additional topping suggestions (optional):

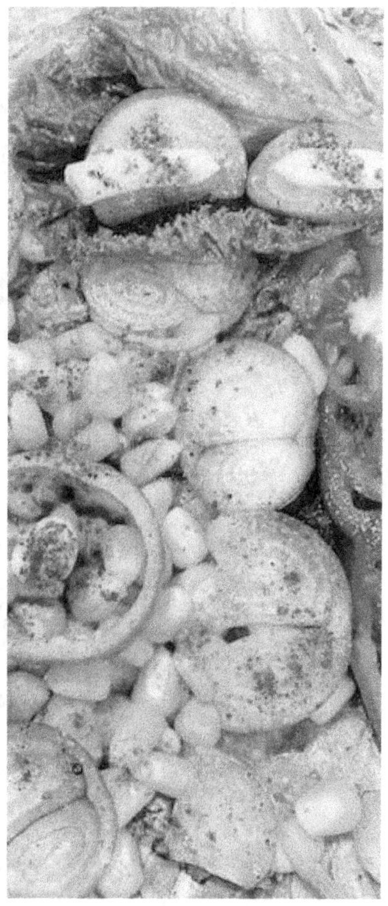

Pickled jalapeño, queso fresco or feta cheese, roasted pepitas

Directions:

- Set the oven to 425°F. Add sweet potatoes to a big sheet pan (you may use parchment paper if you'd like, but it's not required).

- Add a drizzle of olive oil and season with one tablespoon of chili powder and approximately one teaspoon of salt. Toss to coat. Roast sweet potatoes for 25 to 30 minutes, stirring them halfway through or until soft and lightly browned. While the rice is heating, add a tablespoon of olive oil and a generous amount of salt to the saucepan and cook the rice as directed on the box.

- Stir in the cilantro and lime zest once the rice has cooked. If necessary, taste and add additional salt.

- Sprinkle the avocados with some salt and half of the lime juice. Adjust spices according to taste. Set aside to serve.

- In a small bowl, combine the sour cream and chili-lime crema. Incorporate the remaining lime juice, the remaining ½ teaspoon of chili powder, a few dashes of hot sauce, and a little salt. After tasting, adjust the seasonings. Set aside for serving.

- Scoop sweet potatoes, black beans, avocado, bell peppers, and a drizzle of crema over the rice in bowls; add more toppings if you'd like.

Nutritional Information:

Calories: 380

Protein: 10g

Fiber: 12g

Healthy Fats: 15g

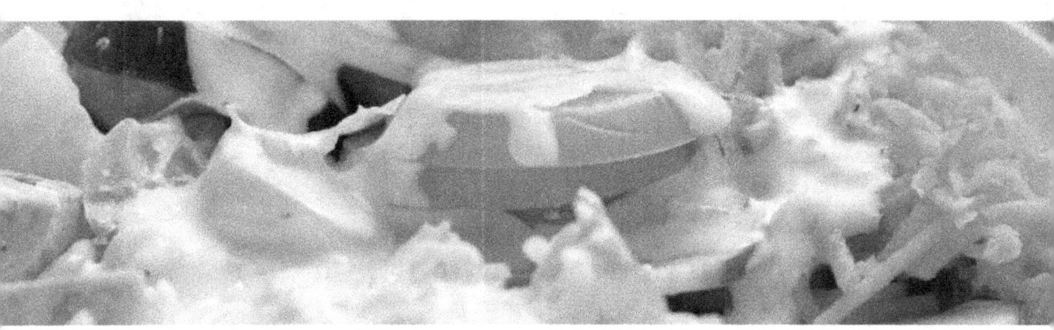

Quinoa-chickpea salad with tomatoes and lemon-tahini dressing

Total time: 30 Minutes   Number of Servings 2

Ingredients

½ cup rainbow quinoa

2 tablespoons currants

2 tablespoons sherry vinegar

1 cup cooked chickpeas

1 summer squash

3 tablespoons roasted almonds

Mediterranean spice blend
(sumac - coriander-cumin)

⅓ Cup peas

1 cucumber

2½ ounces cherry tomatoes

1 lemon

Fresh mint

2 ounces of baby arugula

Sun basket lemon-tahini dressing
(tahini - fresh garlic - lemon juice
- salt)

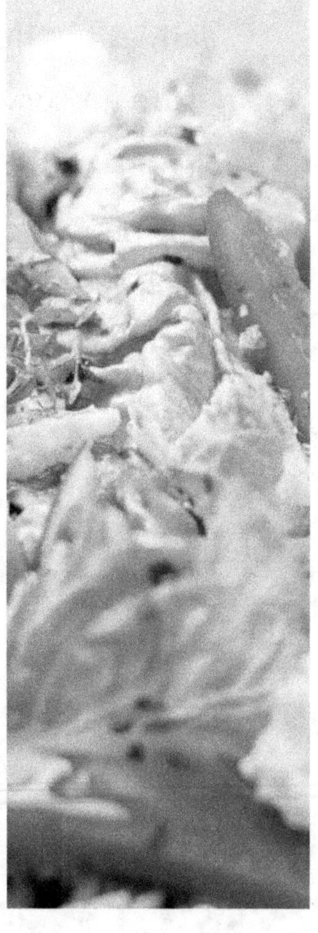

Directions

- Rinse the quinoa in a fine-mesh sieve.

- Quinoa and one cup of gently salted water should be combined in a small saucepan. Once the quinoa is soft and the water has been absorbed, cook it for 15 to 20 minutes on high heat, then lower the heat to a simmer and cover.

- As the quinoa is cooking, prepare the squash, chickpeas, and currants.

- The currants and sherry vinegar should be combined in a separate dish and left to soak until you're ready to mix the salad.

- Rinse the chickpeas.

- Summer squash should have its ends cut off before being sliced half lengthwise and crosswise into thin half-moons.

- Chop the almonds coarsely.

- Heat one or two tablespoons of oil in a big skillet over medium-high heat until it's hot but not smoking.

- Add the almonds, squash, chickpeas, and Mediterranean spice mixture and Cook, stirring often, for 2 to 3 minutes or until the squash is soft. Take off the heat and mix in the peas. Use salt and pepper to season to taste.

- As the squash cooks, prepare the other ingredients for the salad.

- If desired, peel the cucumber and cut off the ends. Cut in half lengthwise, then in half crosswise to form half-moons ¼ inch thick.

- Cut the cherry tomatoes in half.

- Juice half of the lemon, then cut the other half into wedges to decorate.

- Strip the mint leaves from their stems and roughly cut them.

- The arugula, quinoa, cucumber, tomatoes, lemon juice, mint, and the chickpea-squash combination should all be combined in a medium-sized bowl. Incorporate the currants into the salad using a slotted spoon. Add salt and pepper to taste, then toss thoroughly to coat.

- Serve

- Spoon the salad into separate dishes. Present the lemon wedges and the dressing with lemon tahini separately.

- Make It Leaner: Our tahini dressing packs a lot of calories despite being tasty and healthy. You may cut down on 12 grams of fat and 145 calories by using only 1 tablespoon of dressing. Moreover, you'll have plenty to use later as a vegetable dip. Try diluting the dressing with a small amount of water to boost its volume without adding extra calories.

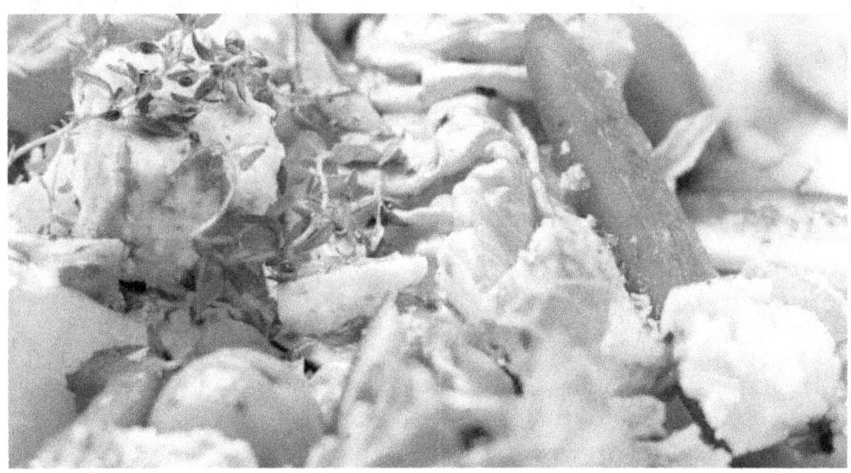

CHAPTER SIX

Chickpea and Vegetable Stir Fry

Total time: 15 Minutes   Number of Servings 4

Ingredients:

For the sauce:

½ cup water

¼-1/2 cup soy sauce or tamari

2 tablespoons coconut or cane sugar

2 teaspoons cornstarch

Sriracha sauce to taste

Vegetables:

½ red onion, julienned

½ red bell pepper, julienned

8 Brussels sprouts, quartered

1 15-ounce can of chickpeas, drained

Sesame seeds, optional

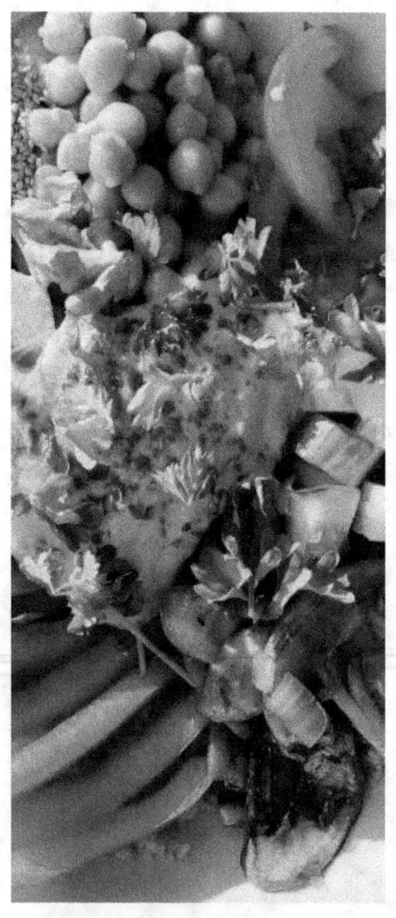

Directions

- Transfer some boiling water to a pan and sauté the vegetables for one to two minutes on high heat. After draining, put them aside.
- After putting all the sauce components in the wok, simmer them for five minutes over medium-high heat or until the sauce thickens.
- After adding the vegetables and chickpeas, cook for an additional two minutes over medium-high heat.
- Sprinkle some sesame seeds on top and serve.

Nutritional Information

Calories: 234kcal

Carbohydrates: 32.9g

Protein: 7.6g

Fat: 1.3g

Spaghetti with lentil Bolognese

Total time: 20 Minutes   Number of Servings 4

Ingredients:

400g spaghetti

2 tbsp olive oil

1 onion, finely chopped

1 celery stalk, finely chopped

3 garlic cloves, finely chopped

420g jar cherry tomato pasta sauce (see note)

250g punnet cherry tomatoes

400g can lentils, rinsed and drained

1/2 cup (40g) grated vegetarian hard cheese (or parmesan)

Basil leaves to serve

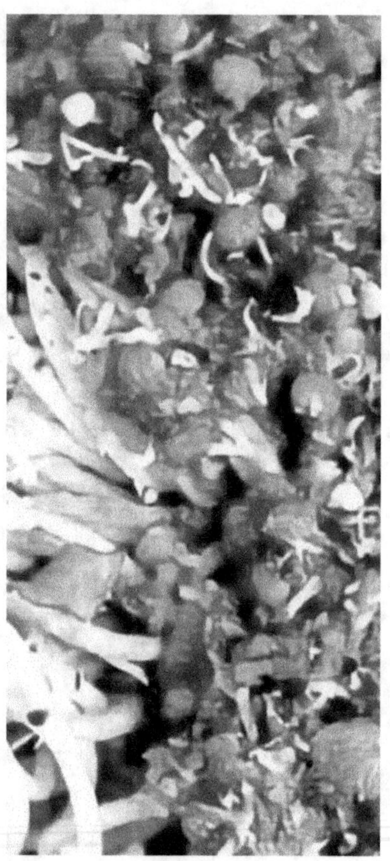

Directions

- As directed on the package, cook the pasta in a big pot of boiling salted water.

- In the meantime, soften the onion, celery, and garlic for two minutes by heating the oil in a frying pan over medium heat.

- After adding the spaghetti sauce and 1/2 cup (125 ml) water, Simmer and cook the tomatoes for five minutes or until they become tender. Cook for a further minute after adding the lentils and seasoning.

- After draining, combine spaghetti with sauce. Spoon into individual bowls and garnish with basil leaves and vegan hard cheese or parmesan.

Nutritional Information

Calories: 234kcal

Carbohydrates: 32.9g

Protein: 7.6g

Fat: 1.3g

Stuffed Bell Peppers with Quinoa and Black Beans

Total time: 1 hours

Number of Servings 4

Ingredients:

4 large bell peppers, de-seeded; tops cut and chopped for the filling; the peppers cut in half lengthwise to hold the filling

2 cups cooked quinoa

1 cup canned black beans, drained and rinsed

1 cup pasta sauce (I used roasted garlic flavor)

¼ cup cilantro, coarsely chopped, plus more for topping

½ cup cheddar cheese, plus more for topping

Salt and pepper to taste

Optional: sour cream or Greek yogurt as topping

Directions

- Set the oven to 350 degrees Fahrenheit. Using parchment paper, line a 9 x 13 baking pan.

- As directed on the package, prepare the quinoa.

- Combine the cooked quinoa, black beans, cheese, spaghetti sauce, chopped bell pepper tops, cilantro, salt, and pepper in a big bowl.

- Place the filling inside each bell pepper. Put the peppers in the baking dish side by side, cover with aluminum foil, and bake for 25 to 30 minutes or until the peppers are soft.

- Garnish with more cheese, cilantro, sour cream, or Greek yogurt if desired. Serve right away.

Nutritional Information

Calories: 234kcal

Carbohydrates: 32.9g

Protein: 7.6g

Fat: 1.3g

Roasted Veggie and Hummus Wrap

Total time: 35minutes   Number of Servings 6

Ingredients

6 whole meal tortilla wraps (whole wheat wraps)

1 medium sweet potato

1 red pepper

1 zucchini

2 tablespoon harissa paste

6 tablespoon hummus

1 cup fresh baby spinach

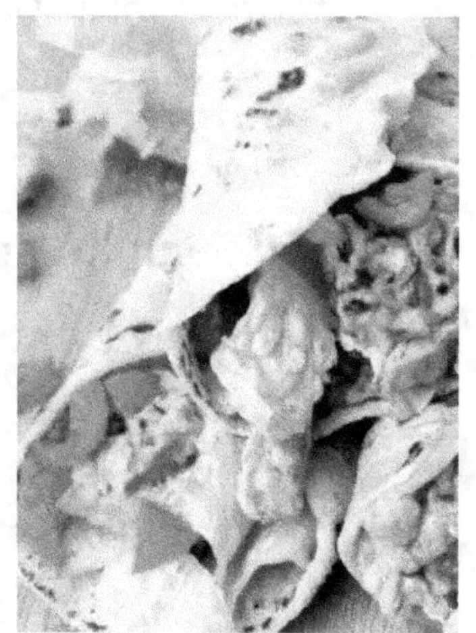

Directions:

- Preheat the oven to 390 degrees Fahrenheit (200 degrees Celsius).

- Peel and chop the sweet potato, zucchini, and red pepper into tiny pieces.

- Toss well after adding the harissa paste.

- After moving the veggies to a pan, bake them for 20 to 25 minutes or until soft.

- Top a tortilla wrap with a tablespoon of hummus, baby spinach, and roughly a tablespoon of roasted vegetables. Make sure the edges stay tight as you wrap.

Repeat with the remaining ingredients.

Nutritional Information

Calories: 194kcal

Carbohydrates: 32g

Protein: 6g

Fat: 4g

Cauliflower and Chickpea Curry

Total time: 25minutes   Number of Servings 2-4

Ingredients:

1 medium cauliflower (around 4 cups)

1 tin/400g chickpeas, drained

1 red onion

4 garlic cloves

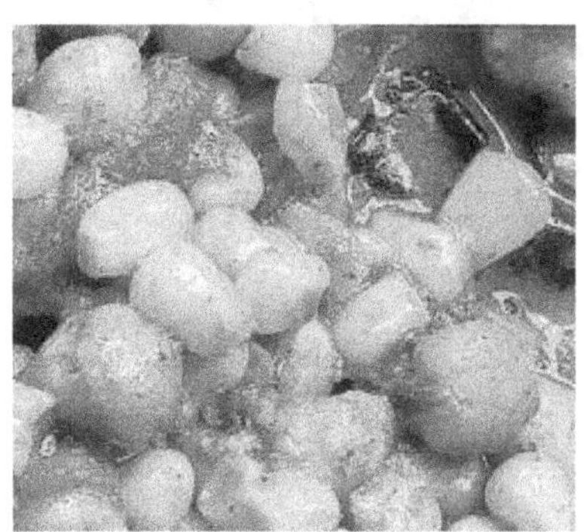

Inch of ginger

1 tbsp curry powder, medium

1 tsp ground cumin

1/2 tsp garam masala

1/4 tsp ground turmeric

1/4 tsp chilli powder

1/4 tsp salt

1 tin/400g tinned chopped tomatoes

1 tbsp tomato puree

1 tin/400ml full-fat coconut milk

Optional toppings:

Drizzle of vegan cream

Fresh coriander

1/2 cup/120ml vegetable

Directions

- Warm up a tablespoon of oil in a big pan over medium heat.

- After a few minutes, add the finely chopped onion and continue to simmer. Finally, stir in the grated ginger and garlic.

- Stirring often to prevent burning, cook for one minute.

- Add the salt, turmeric, chili powder, garam masala, cumin, and curry powder. Simmer for about 30 seconds or until aromatic. If it's too dry, add a bit of extra oil.

- Add the tomato puree and diced tomatoes. Cook for a few minutes while stirring.

- Once smooth, transfer to a bowl, puree with a hand blender or in a blender, and then put back in the pan.

- Add the cauliflower, stock, and coconut milk. Bite-sized chunks of cauliflower should be cut; they shouldn't be too big or too little.

- After 10 to 15 minutes of simmering, add the chickpeas and cook for an additional five minutes.

- Although mushy, the cauliflower should still have some bite to it. Cook it for a little longer if you want it tender.

- Add some fresh coriander and coconut milk or vegan cream as garnish!

Nutritional Information

Calories: 596

Carbohydrates: 57g

Protein: 20g

Fat: 36g

Mushroom and Spinach Stuffed Portobello Mushrooms

Total time: 40 minutes   Number of Servings 4

Ingredients:

4 Portobello mushrooms

1/2 lb. frozen spinach

1/2 cup cottage cheese

1/2 cup shredded mozzarella

2 oz. feta

1 large egg

1/4 tsp garlic powder

1/8 tsp salt

1/8 tsp freshly cracked black pepper

1/8 tsp crushed red pepper

1 Tbsp. olive oil ($0.16)

1/2 cup marinara sauce (optional)

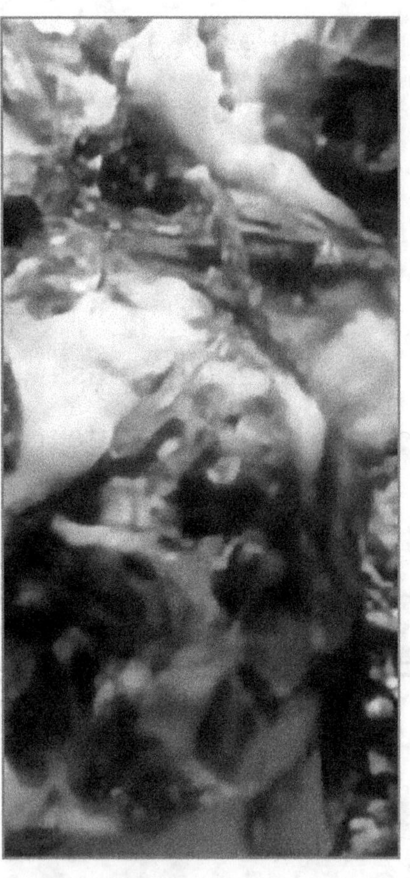

Directions.

- Set oven temperature to 400°F. After thawing the frozen spinach, remove as much water as you can.

- Squeezed spinach, cottage cheese, mozzarella, feta, egg, garlic powder, salt, pepper, and crushed red pepper should all be combined in a bowl. Mix until all ingredients are well blended.

- Make sure to clean the Portobello mushrooms of any dirt or debris. Take the stems off. Sprinkle a small amount of salt and oil on top of the mushroom caps for seasoning.

- Arrange the mushrooms on a baking sheet, gill side up. Spoon the filling of cheese and spinach among the four mushrooms, packing it firmly into the caps.

- The cheese mixture on top should softly brown after 25 minutes of baking the stuffed Portobello mushrooms in a preheated oven. Since mushrooms are high in water, it is expected to observe liquid leaking from them.

- Top each spinach-stuffed Portobello with two tablespoons of marinara sauce before serving.

Nutritional Information

Calories: 207.78kcal

Carbohydrates: 9.68g

Protein: 14.03g

Fat: 12.8g

Quinoa Salad with Avocado and Lime Dressing

Total time: 35 minutes   Number of Servings 2-3

Ingredients:

1 cup (cooked) quinoa

1/2 cup canned black beans, drained and rinsed

1/2 cup frozen corn (thawed)

1/2 of a bell pepper, diced

1/2 cup cherry tomatoes, halved

2 tbsp red onion, diced

1 tbsp cilantro, chopped (optional)

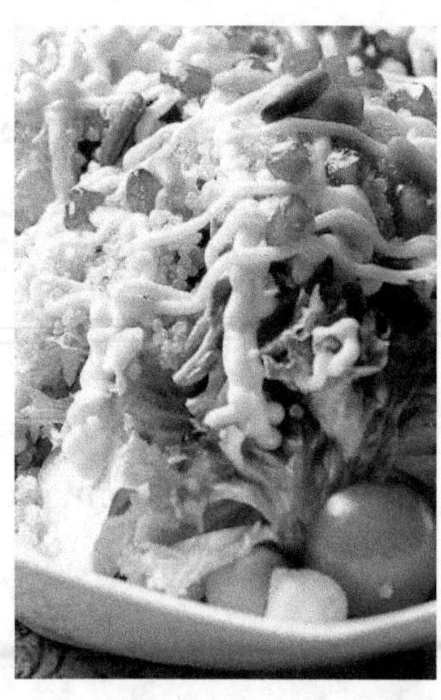

1 avocado, cubed

1/4 cup feta cheese

For the dressing:

1 tbsp olive oil

2 tbsp fresh lime juice

1/2 tsp honey

1/4 tsp garlic powder

Salt + pepper, to taste

Optional: Splash of hot sauce for a spicy dressing

Directions;

- As directed on the package, prepare the quinoa.

- The cooked quinoa should be well combined with the black beans, corn, tomatoes, red onion, bell pepper, and cilantro in a big dish.

- Mix thoroughly after adding the dressing.

- Fold in the diced avocado* gently, and then top with feta. Serve and savor after tasting and adding extra salt and pepper as needed. It can be prepped ahead for up to 3 days.

Nutritional Information

Calories: 270

Protein: 6g

Fiber: 8g

Vitamin C: 25%

Sweet Potato and Black Bean Enchiladas

Total time: 1 hr. 10 mins   Number of Servings 5

Ingredients:

Red Enchilada Sauce:

2 tablespoons vegetable oil

2 cloves garlic, minced

1 1/2 cups tomato sauce

3/4 cup reduced-sodium chicken broth

1/2 teaspoon chipotle chile powder

1/2 teaspoon ground cumin

1 to 3 chipotle chiles in adobo sauce, chopped

Kosher salt and freshly ground black pepper

Enchilada Filling:

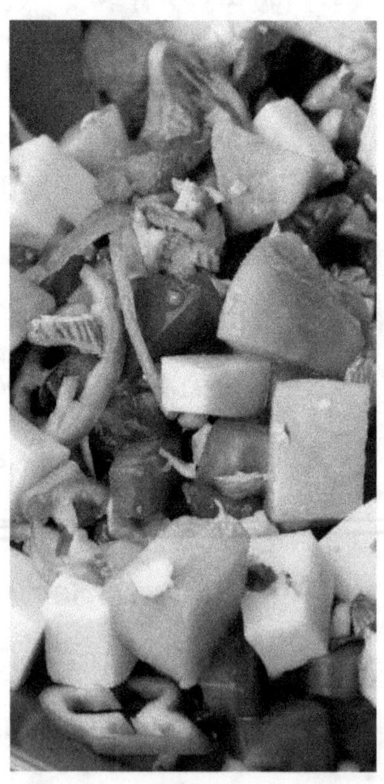

1 cup red enchilada sauce,

Homemade or canned

(Recipe above)

1 teaspoon olive oil

3 cloves garlic, minced

1 small onion, diced

1 jalapeño, seeded and diced

2 1/2 cups sweet potatoes (about 1 large), peeled and cut into 1/2-inch cubes

One 10-ounce can of diced tomatoes with green chiles, such as Rotel

1 1/2 cups canned reduced-sodium black beans, rinsed and drained

1/4 cup fresh cilantro, plus more for garnishing

1 teaspoon ground cumin

1/2 teaspoon chili powder

Kosher salt and freshly ground black pepper

Assembly:

10 medium low-carb whole-wheat flour tortillas, such as La Tortilla Factory

2 cups reduced-fat shredded Mexican cheese

Reduced-fat sour cream for serving, optional

Directions:

- Before baking, preheat the oven to 400°F. Line the bottom of a 13 by 9-inch baking dish with 1/4 cup red enchilada sauce.

- In a large pan, heat the olive oil over medium-high heat. Add the garlic, onions, and jalapeño and simmer for approximately 2 minutes until the garlic is aromatic and the onions turn translucent.

- Add chopped tomatoes, black beans, cilantro, cumin, chili powder, cubed sweet potatoes, and 1/4 cup of water. After covering and cooking for about ten minutes over medium-low heat, stirring now and again, the sweet potatoes should be soft.

- Fill each tortilla to the brim with a full 1/3 cup of filling, roll it up, and set seam-side down in the baking dish.

- Add the cheese and the remaining 3/4 cup of enchilada sauce over top.

- Bake the enchiladas for approximately ten minutes, covered with foil, or until they are heated and the cheese has melted. If preferred, top with more cilantro and serve with sour cream.

- Add the oil to a medium saucepan set over medium-low heat, and sauté the garlic for approximately 30 seconds or until fragrant. Stir in the chipotle chilies, cumin, tomato sauce, chicken broth, and a dash of salt and pepper. Heat till boiling.

- Reduce the heat to low and simmer for 5 to 7 minutes or until the mixture thickens slightly. Set aside until you're ready to utilize it.

Nutritional Information

Calories: 207.78kcal

Carbohydrates: 9.68g

Protein: 14.03g

Fat: 12.8g

Vegan Lentil Soup

Total time: 1 hr. Number of Servings 6

Ingredients:

1 ½ cups chopped yellow onions

1 cup chopped carrots

3 cloves garlic, minced

2 tablespoons extra-virgin olive oil

2 tablespoons no-salt-added tomato paste

4 cups of reduced-sodium vegetable broth

1 cup water

1 (15 ounces) can no-salt-added cannellini beans, rinsed

1 cup mixed dry lentils (brown, green, and black)

½ cup chopped sun-dried tomatoes in oil drained

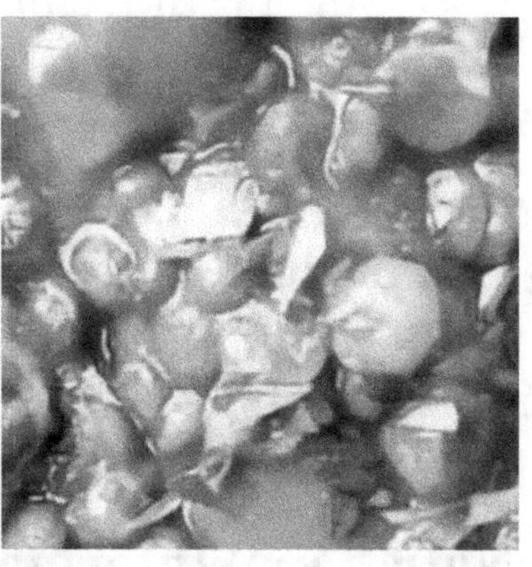

¾ teaspoon salt

½ teaspoon ground pepper

1 tablespoon chopped fresh dill, plus more for garnish

1 ½ teaspoons red wine vinegar

Directions

- In a big, heavy saucepan, heat the oil over medium heat. Add the onions and carrots and simmer, stirring regularly, for 3 to 4 minutes or until softened.

- Add the garlic and simmer for approximately a minute, stirring frequently, until fragrant. When the mixture is uniformly covered, add the tomato paste and simmer, stirring frequently, for about one minute.

- Add the lentils, cannellini beans, sun-dried tomatoes, broth, water, salt, and pepper and stir. Over medium-high heat, bring to a boil; lower heat to medium-low to keep simmering.

- Cover and simmer for 30 to 40 minutes or until the lentils are soft.

- Take off the heat and mix in the vinegar and dill. If desired, garnish with more dill and serve.

Nutritional Information

Calories: 272

Carbohydrates: 42g

Protein: 13g

Fat: 7g

Stir-Fried Tofu with Broccoli and Teriyaki Sauce

Total time: 30 Minutes   Number of Servings 4

Ingredients:

4 cups cooked rice

1 medium white onion, sliced thinly

3 tablespoons canola oil, divided

1 14-ounce block of Simple Truth firm tofu

2 broccoli crowns, chopped (about 4 cups)

¼ cup water

1 cup Private Selection Mukimame beans, thawed

1 cup Private Selection Sesame Teriyaki Stir Fry Sauce

¼ cup chopped green onion

Sesame seeds

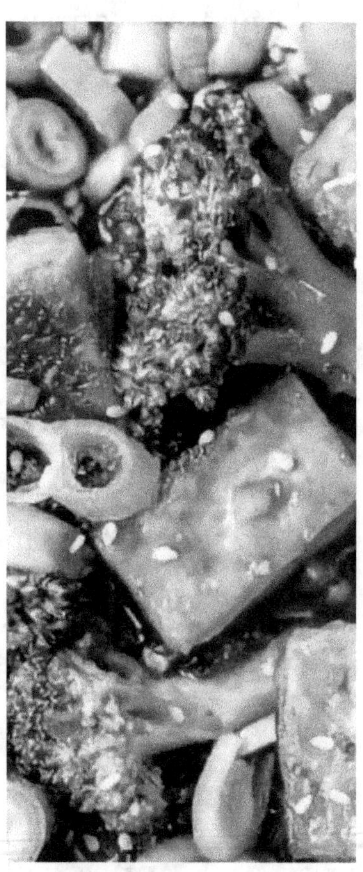

Directions

- To begin with, drain the tofu by placing one folded paper towel below it on a dish and another folded paper towel on top of it. To extract the liquid from the tofu, place another plate on top of it and weigh it down with a bowl filled with something heavy.

- After ten minutes, swap out the paper towels halfway through the draining process. Cut the tofu into small pieces and save.

- Over high heat, preheat a wok or nonstick skillet. To the wok, add two teaspoons of canola oil. Add the tofu after the oil begins to ripple. Cook the tofu in batches, stirring occasionally, for 3–4 minutes until the underside is crisp and golden. Then, gently flip the tofu with tongs or chopsticks to brown the other side. Place the cooked tofu onto a paper towel-lined platter.

- Add the onion to the wok after heating the remaining oil. Stir-fry for two to three minutes, then add the broccoli and slowly pour in ¼ cup of water, being careful not to let it splash. Stir-fry for 2 to 3 minutes or until the broccoli is crisp-tender.

- Stir-fry the tofu and Mikimame beans in the pan with the teriyaki sauce after frying for another three to four minutes. Serve over rice and garnish with sesame seeds and scallions.

Nutritional Information

Calories: 615kcal

Carbohydrates: 85g

Protein: 31g

Fat: 19g

CHAPTER SEVEN

Smoothies and Juices Recipes

Green Goddess Smoothie

Total time: 5 Minutes   Number of Servings 2

Ingredients:

2 green apples

2 cups almond milk

1 banana (frozen preferred)

2 cups kale or spinach

4 Tablespoons peanut butter

2 Tablespoons flaxseeds

2 Tablespoons maple syrup

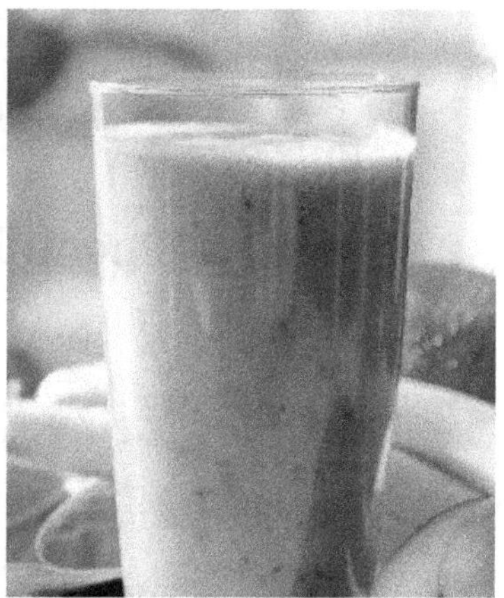

Directions

- Just fill your high-powered blender with almond milk, peanut butter, flaxseeds, maple syrup, and all your prepped fruits and veggies. Blend the ingredients until it becomes creamy and thick. Transfer into cups or glasses and enjoy!

- You may experiment with adding more water, fruit juice, or almond milk if you want your smoothies to be thinner.

- Try freezing your apple and greens before blending them, or add a frozen banana if you want your smoothies thicker. A handful of ice is an excellent backup plan in case everything fails.

- Make a smoothie bowl out of it! Use as little liquid as possible to achieve this. Fill the blender with all the ingredients (except the almond milk) and add one spoonful of almond milk at a time while the blender is blending. Proceed until your smoothie reaches a thick and smooth consistency suitable for spoon-feeding.

Variations

A vegan kale smoothie may be easily tailored to your nutritional requirements and preferences. Next time, consider including any of the following ideas:

Greens: Try to include arugula, spinach, micro greens, or Swiss chard to boost your vitamin intake.

Fruit: To get a creamy texture, freeze avocado chunks. Adding strawberries, blueberries, and blackberries to this smoothie will also make it sweet, nutrient-dense, and delightful.

Liquid: Feel free to substitute your preferred milk for this smoothie if almond or dairy-free milk isn't your thing. Instead of milk, substitute water or fruit juice, such as orange or apple juice.

Add-ins: Increase the amount of nut butter or your preferred protein powder to increase the protein content. Goji berries, cacao nibs, and cinnamon may all contribute sweetness and a variety of tastes.

Nutritional Information

Calories: 510kcal

Carbohydrates: 68g

Protein: 15g

Fat: 3g

Blueberry Bliss Smoothie

| Total time: 5 Minutes | Number of Servings 2 |

Ingredients

1 cup / 200 g / frozen blueberry

1 cup / 150 g / frozen strawberry

3/4 cup / 170 g / frozen banana

1 cup / 240 ml/milk of choice (dairy or non-dairy; I used almond milk)

1 tbsp maple syrup

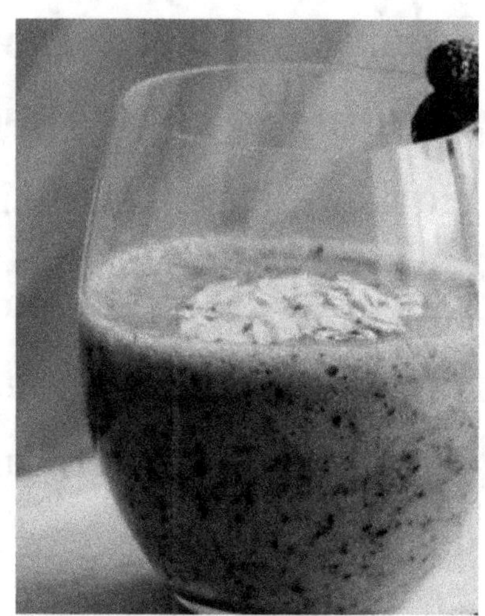

Directions

- Add liquids. Transfer the milk and maple syrup to the bottom of a high-powdered blender.

- Add frozen fruit. The frozen blueberries, strawberries, and banana slices should be layered on top. Add any other ingredients, such as nuts or seeds, if you'd like.

- Blend. Mix all the ingredients in a blender for one to two minutes or until extremely smooth and creamy.

- Serve. Pour the smoothie between two glasses, and feel free to top with some strawberries and blueberries. Savor it immediately!

Nutritional Information

Calories: 246

Carbohydrates: 53g

Protein: 15g

Fat: 6g

Turmeric Citrus Juice

Total time: 5 Minutes   Number of Servings 1

Ingredients

2 Fuji apples, cored and sliced

1 orange, peeled and sectioned

½ lemon, peeled

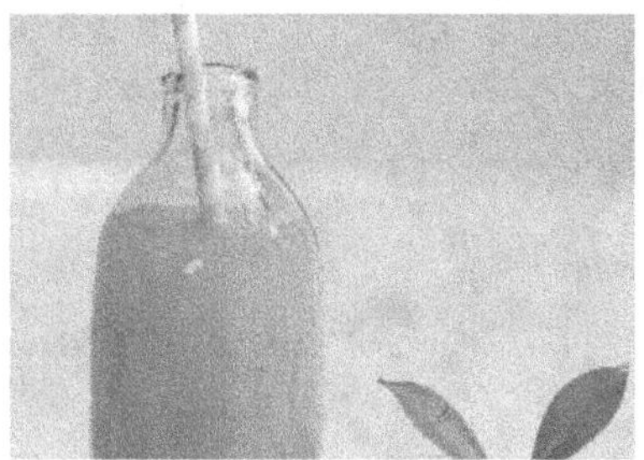

Directions

- Juice the apples, orange, lemon, and ginger; mix in the turmeric until well combined.

Nutritional Information

Calories: 163

Carbohydrates: 46g

Protein: 2g

Fat: 1g

Anti-Oxidant Powerhouse Smoothie

Total time: 3 Minutes   Number of Servings 1

Ingredients

3/4 cup Nature's Promise® Organic Berry Medley

1/4 cup plain nonfat Greek yogurt

3/4 cup Nature's Promise® 100% Pomegranate Juice

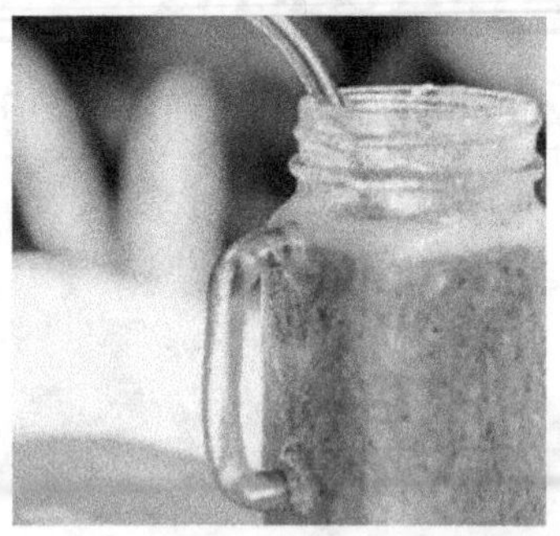

Direction

Blend all ingredients until smooth in a blender. Pour into a glass and serve.

Nutritional Information

Calories: 230kcal

Carbohydrates: 46.0g

Protein: 8.0g

Fat: 3.0g

Carrot Ginger Zinger Juice

Total time: 4 minutes   Number of Servings 1

Ingredients

1 frozen sliced ripe banana

1/2 cup unsweetened applesauce

1/2 cup non-fat plain Greek yogurt

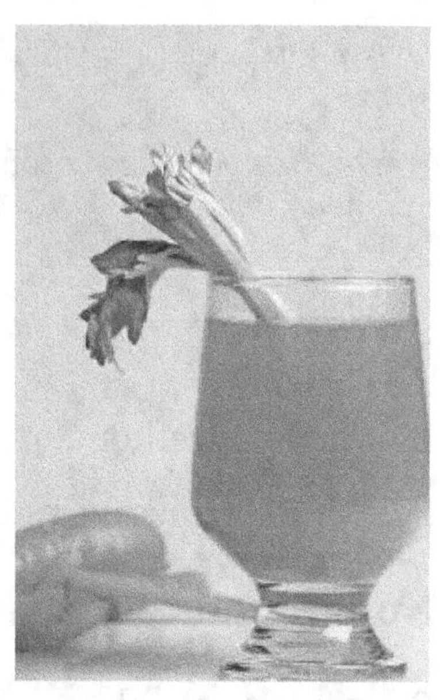

Directions

- In a blender, combine all the ingredients and process until smooth. Serve right away.

Nutritional Information

Calories: 230kcal

Carbohydrates: 46.0g

Protein: 8.0g

Fat: 3.0g

Total time: 10 minutes   Number of Servings 1

Ingredients

Drink:

3 cucumber

1 lemon, juiced

1/2 tsp. lemon zest

5-8 sprigs mint

2 tbsp. honey, or agave, or sugar syrup, to taste

1-inch ginger

1/2 tsp black salt

1/4 tsp. salt

1 bottle of carbonated water or soda

Garnish:

1 cucumber

1 lemon

1 1/2 tsp chaat masala

1/2 tsp red chili powder

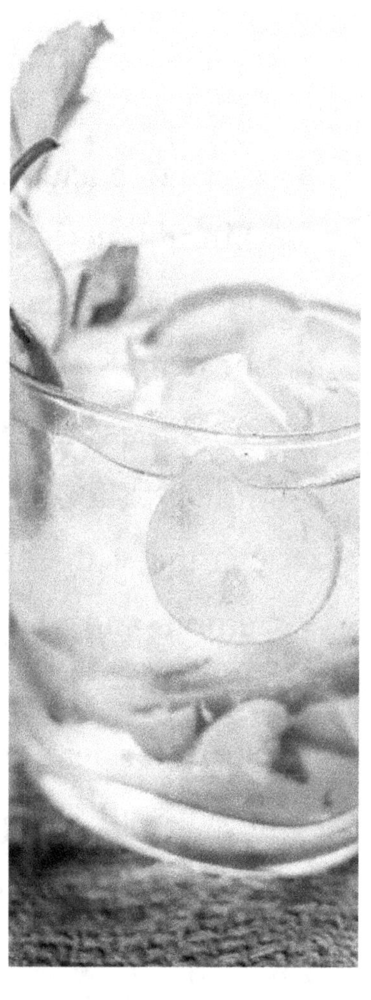

Directions

- Put the peeled cucumbers, ginger, lemon zest, juice, mint, black salt, and sweetener in a blender. Blend till smooth, then taste and adjust to your preference. This drink can also be kept in the refrigerator if it will be served later.

- Another cucumber can be shaved or sliced into thin ribbons lengthwise. Another lemon should be cut into slices. Keep both of them aside for the drink's garnish.

- Combine your chili powder and chaat masala in a dish to form the rim garnish. To get a good coating, rub the rims of your glasses with a lemon and then dip them into the masala mixture.

- Slices of lemon, cucumber ribbons, and ice should all be added to your glass. Pour the cucumber juice halfway into them, then cover with soda or fizzy water. Enjoy your dish and garnish it with a second slice of lemon dipped in masala!

Nutritional Information

Calories: 51

Carbohydrates: 14g

Protein: 1g

Fat: 1g

Pomegranate Green Tea Smoothie

Total time: 10 minutes   Number of Servings 1

Ingredients

Pomegranate Green Tea Ingredients:

4 cups hot water

4 green tea bags or about 4 teaspoons of leaf green tea in a strainer or filter

4 tablespoons grenadine

Grenadine Ingredients:

1 cup 100% pomegranate juice

1 cup sugar

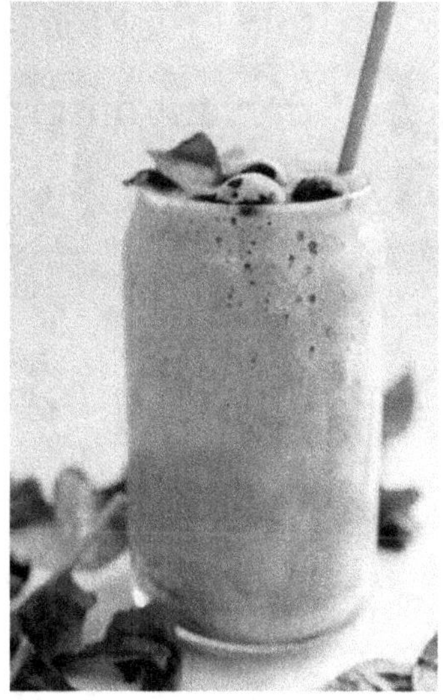

Direction

Make your grenadine first. In a saucepan, combine sugar and pomegranate juice in equal parts and heat. Until the sugar dissolves completely, stir. Transfer to a jar.

- Bring your water to a near-boiling temperature using a kettle or stovetop.
- Transfer into a pitcher or quart jar. Include loose tea leaves or tea bags. For 60 seconds, brew to prevent bitterness. After a few dips, take the tea bags out of the jar. Again, to prevent bitterness, do not press the tea bags.
- When adding grenadine, stir. Let cool or serve chilled over ice!

Nutritional Information

Calories: 20.4 kcal

Carbohydrates: 5 g

Protein: 0.1g

Fat: 0.1g

Golden Glow Turmeric Smoothie

Total time: 5 minutes   Number of Servings 2

Ingredients

½ cup full-fat coconut milk

¼ cup collagen peptides

½ teaspoon turmeric powder

Pinch freshly ground pepper.

1 small frozen banana cut into coins

1 Persian or Armenian seedless cucumber 6-inches, cut into coins

1 cup frozen mango chunks

Honey maple syrup or stevia to taste (optional)

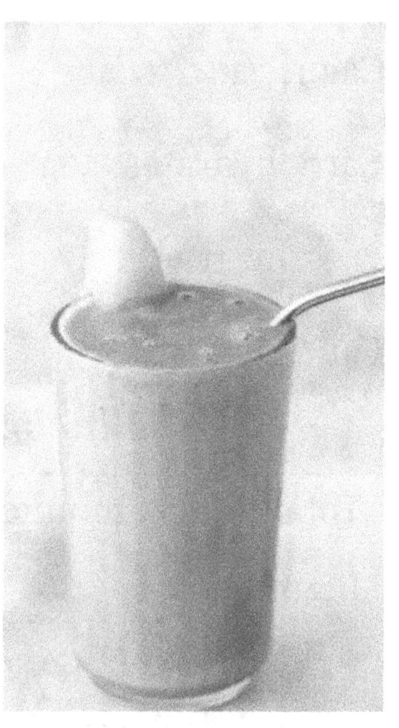

Direction

- Add the mango, banana, cucumber, collagen peptides, turmeric, freshly ground pepper, and coconut milk. You may now add more sweetness if you'd like.

- Blend until smooth!

- Either divide it between two glasses or consume it all at once!

Nutritional Information

Calories: 271kcal

Carbohydrates: 27g

Protein: 17g

Fat: 12g

Blueberry Kale Elixir

Total time: 5 minutes   Number of Servings 2

Ingredients

1 ½ cups cold coconut water

2 cups lightly packed kale, roughly chopped

2 cups frozen wild blueberries

1 orange peeled and cut in half

1 tablespoon flax seeds

2 Brazil nuts

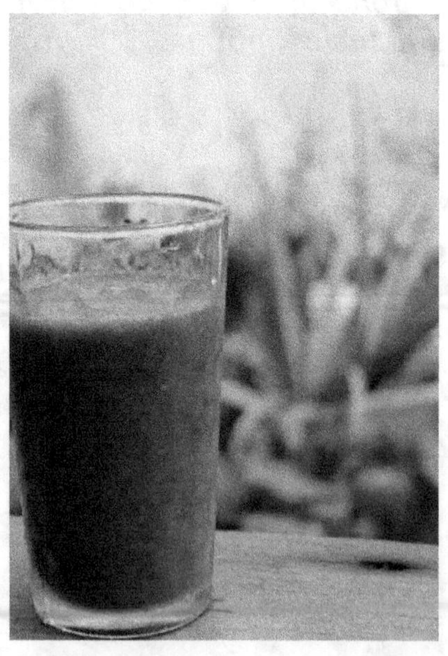

Direction

- Blend the ingredients in a blender until they are smooth.
- Transfer into a glass and serve immediately, or refrigerate for up to one hour.

Nutritional Information

Calories: 271kcal

Carbohydrates: 27g

Protein: 17g

Fat: 12g

Mango Matcha Smoothie

Total time: 10 minutes   Number of Servings 2

Ingredients

1 ½" piece ginger, peeled, finely grated

1¾ cups frozen cubed mango

1 cup plain whole-milk yogurt

2 teaspoons matcha (green tea powder)

1 teaspoon vanilla extract

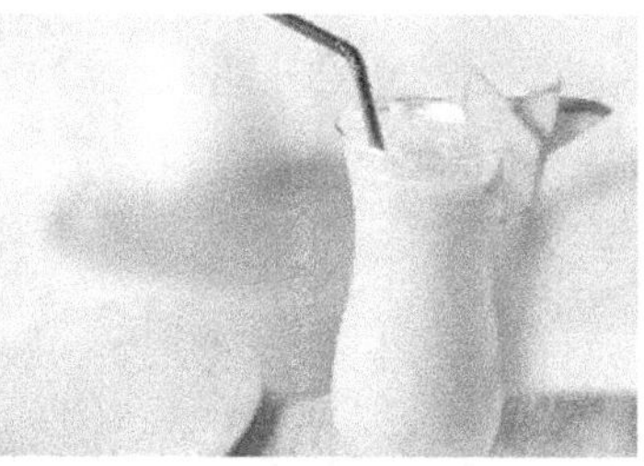

½ teaspoon agave syrup (optional)

Directional

Blend the ginger, mango, yogurt, matcha, vanilla, and agave syrup (if desired) with ½ cup cool water until smooth, and then distribute among glasses.

Nutritional Information

Calories: 271kcal

Carbohydrates: 27g

Protein: 17g

Fat: 12g

Roasted Brussels sprouts

Total time: 30 minutes   Number of Servings 4

Ingredients

1/2 teaspoon kosher salt

1/4 teaspoon black pepper

1 tablespoon, plus 1 teaspoon extra-virgin olive oil

1 1/2 pounds Brussels sprouts, trimmed and halved

Optional flavor additions

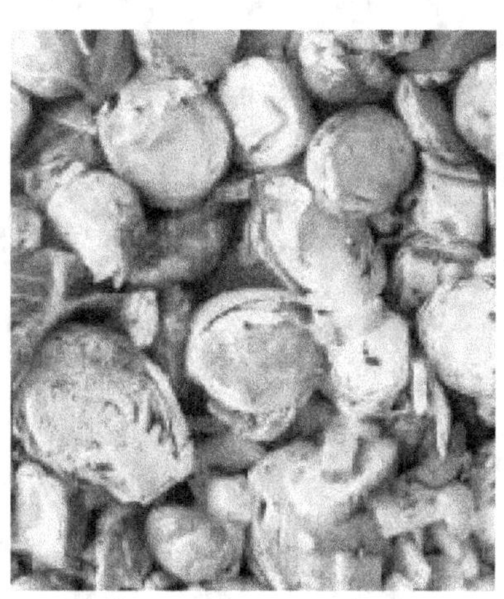

Direction

- Set an oven rack in the top third of the oven and warm to 400°F.

- Arrange the Brussels sprouts in the middle of a large baking sheet with a rim. After adding a drizzle of olive oil, season with salt, pepper, and any additional spices you'd like. Spread the Brussels sprouts in a single layer on the baking sheet after gently tossing them to cover them. Turn the Brussels sprouts so the cut sides are down for an even crispier texture.

- Bake the Brussels sprouts for 20 to 30 minutes until they are crisp and slightly browned on the exterior and soft in the middle. The outermost leaves will also be a little black. Because the cooking time will vary depending on the size of your sprouts, keep a close eye on them toward the conclusion of the baking period. To taste, add more salt or pepper for seasoning. Savor right now.

Nutritional Information

Calories: 104kcal

Carbohydrates: 15g

Protein: 6g

Fat: 4g

Turmeric Lentil Soup

Total time: 50 minutes   Number of Servings 6

Ingredients

1 tablespoon avocado oil

1 cup chopped onion

1 cup chopped celery

1 cup chopped turnip or potato

2 1/2 cups chopped sweet potato

2 minced garlic cloves

1 teaspoon sea salt

1 teaspoon black pepper

2 teaspoons dried thyme

1 cup green or brown lentils

1 cup red lentils

1 – 2 tablespoons turmeric (I like 2)

1 teaspoon ginger

1 teaspoon cumin

4 cups vegetable broth

2 cups water

1 cup almond milk

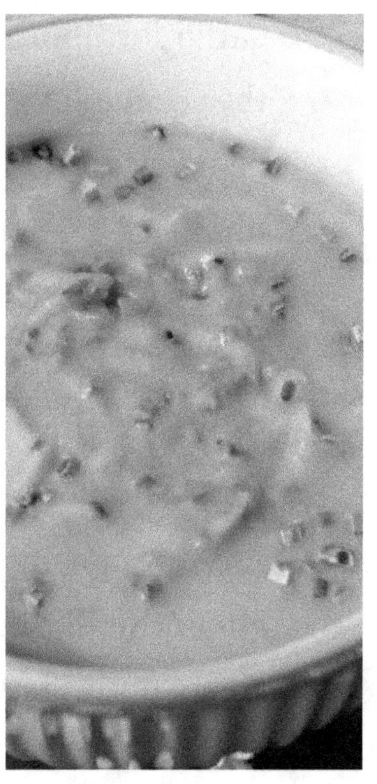

1 cup spinach

1 cup fresh herbs (I like parsley)

1 teaspoon lemon juice

1/2 teaspoon red pepper flakes

Directions

- In a large stockpot or Dutch oven, heat the oil. Saute the turnip, onion, celery, potato, and garlic for approximately five minutes or until the vegetables soften slightly. After adding salt, pepper, and thyme, simmer for about two minutes.

- Add the broth and water after sautéing the lentils for one to two minutes with the turmeric, ginger, and cumin. After boiling the soup, simmer it for 30 minutes while covered.

- After removing from the heat, whisk in the almond milk, herbs, lemon juice, and pepper flakes until the spinach has wilted. Serve right away!

Nutritional Information

Calories: 338kcal

Carbohydrates: 60g

Protein: 18g

Fat: 4g

Roasted Butternut Squash Soup

Total time: 1 hr. 5 mins   Number of Servings 6

Ingredients

1 tablespoon olive oil, plus more for drizzling

½ cup chopped shallot (about 1 large shallot bulb)

1 teaspoon salt

4 garlic cloves, pressed or minced

1 teaspoon maple syrup

⅛ Teaspoon ground nutmeg

Freshly ground black pepper, to taste

1 large butternut squash (about 3 pounds), halved vertically and seeds removed*

3 to 4 cups (24 to 32 ounces) vegetable broth, as needed

1 to 2 tablespoons butter, to taste

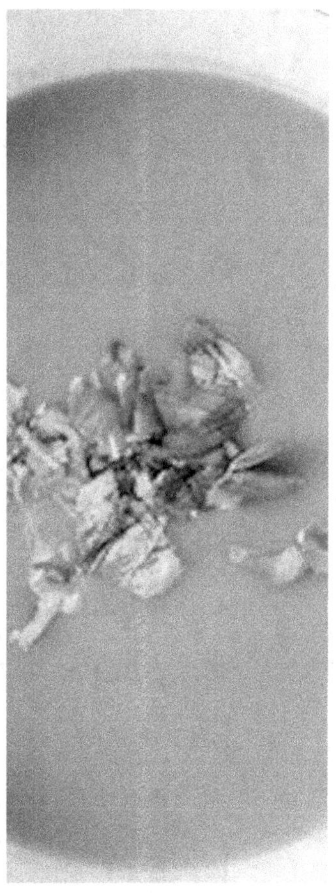

Directions

- Set a baking sheet with parchment paper and preheat the oven to 425°F.

- Scoop each half of the butternut squash into the pan, then season with salt & pepper and ½ teaspoon of olive oil each.
- Roast face down for 40 to 50 minutes or until soft and browned.
- Heat one tablespoon of olive oil in a soup pot. Add one teaspoon of salt, and sauté chopped shallot until golden.
- After adding and cooking the garlic for a minute, transfer it to a blender.
- Remove the peel from the butternut squash and scoop the meat into the blender.
- Add pepper, nutmeg, and maple syrup. Add three cups of veggie broth.
- Blend till very creamy on high speed. Add additional broth as required.
- Pour in the remaining broth to the desired thickness.
- To taste, add one to two tablespoons of butter or olive oil. Well, combine.

- To taste, add salt and pepper for seasoning.

- Transfer to bowls. Warm in the saucepan until steamy, if not hot.

- Add a pinch of black pepper, then savor!

Sweet Potato and Carrot Mash

Total time: 30 minutes   Number of Servings 8

Ingredients

POTATOES & CARROTS

2 medium sweet potatoes, peeled and chopped into large bite-sized pieces

4 medium carrots, peeled and chopped into large bite-sized pieces

Water

THE REST

2-3 Tbsp dairy-free butter (we prefer Miyoko's or Earth Balance // if not vegan, sub organic dairy butter)

2 cloves garlic, minced

1/4 tsp ground ginger

1/2 tsp ground turmeric

Sea salt to taste

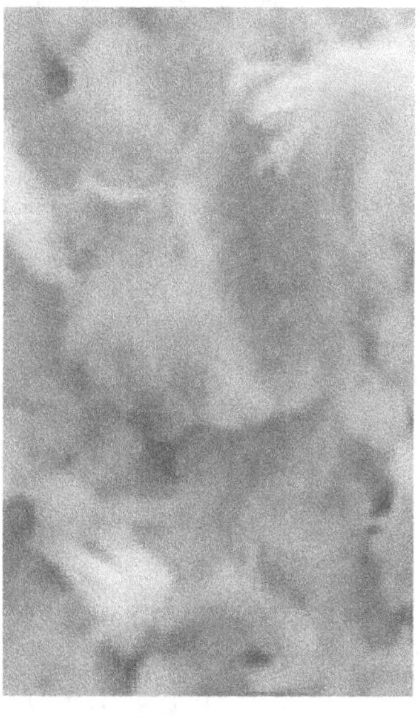

FOR SERVING
optional

Additional butter of choice

Fresh parsley

Salt and pepper

Directions

- Add potatoes and carrots to a large saucepan or Dutch oven after washing, peeling, and chopping them into large, bite-sized pieces. Cover with approximately one inch of water to ensure they're immersed.

- Heat the water to a boiling point. After the potatoes and carrots boil, turn down the heat to medium-high and simmer for another ten to fifteen minutes or until the vegetables are quite soft and easily penetrated with a knife.

- After draining, add the potatoes and carrots to the saucepan (or, for a whipped purée effect, transfer to a food processor or blender). Add your preferred butter, sea salt to taste, minced garlic, ginger, and turmeric. Smoothly mash (or purée). The creamiest texture we discovered was achieved with a food processor. However, mashing also works well, leaving a bit more texture.

- Add a little more water or butter as needed to make it smooth and creamy. If necessary, modify the flavor by adding extra butter for creaminess, spices, or sea salt to taste. Warm up and serve.

- Add salt, pepper, and more butter of your choice as garnish (all optional). Keep refrigerated leftovers for a maximum of four to five days.

Nutritional Information

Calories: 65

Carbohydrates: 9.9g

Protein: 0.9 g

Fat: 2.6 g

Sautéed Garlic Spinach

Total time: 10 minutes   Number of Servings 4

Ingredients

1 pound baby spinach
2 tablespoons olive oil
3 garlic cloves, minced
Salt and pepper, to taste

Direction

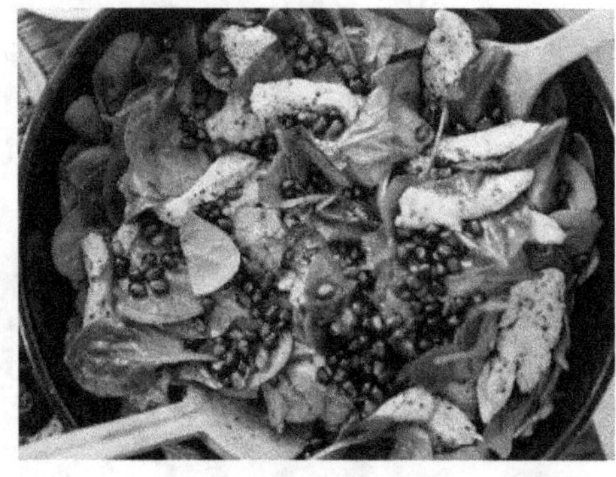

- In a big skillet set over medium-high heat, warm the olive oil. Sauté the minced garlic for 30 seconds after adding it. The garlic shouldn't brown too much.

- Fill the pan with the baby spinach. You may compress it with your hands because it will be a large mound. Toss the spinach over carefully, using tongs or a spatula, so that the oil and garlic coat every piece.

- After a minute of steaming under the cover, stir the pan again. Continue doing this for about five minutes or until the spinach has wilted down.

- Serve after adding salt and pepper for seasoning.

Nutritional Information

Calories: 91kcal65

Carbohydrates: 5g

Protein: 3g

Fat: 7g

Vegetable Stir-Fry with Tofu

Total time: 25minutes   Number of Servings 3

Ingredients

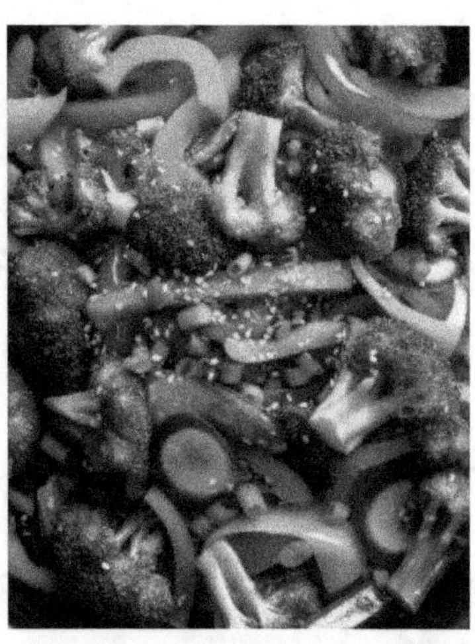

2 (14-ounce) packages of extra-firm tofu do not use firm, silken, or anything other than extra-firm

1 tablespoon canola oil or grape seed oil*

3 tablespoons low-sodium soy sauce divided, plus additional to taste

3 large garlic cloves minced (about 1 heaping tablespoon)

1 small bunch green onions finely chopped, divided

1 tablespoon minced fresh ginger

1–2 teaspoons new chili paste (sambal oelek) or 1/4–1/2 teaspoon red pepper flakes (we like a bit of a kick, so I use the full 2 teaspoons chili paste)

2 teaspoons sesame oil

2 tablespoons toasted sesame seeds

For serving:

Prepared brown rice see Instant Pot Brown Rice

Cauliflower rice

Soba or rice noodles

Quinoa

Directions

- To eliminate extra moisture, wrap each tofu block in two layers of paper towels and carefully wipe dry. Cube the tofu into pieces measuring 3/4 inch.

- Heat canola oil in a large nonstick skillet or wok over medium-high heat. When heated through, gently add the tofu, sprinkle with 1 tablespoon of soy sauce, and cook for 8 to 10 minutes or until browned all over. Stir from time to time so that the tofu gets a good color.

- Stir in the ginger, garlic, most of the green onions, chili paste, and the remaining 2 tablespoons of soy sauce. Cook until aromatic, approximately 1 minute.

- Add handfuls of spinach at a time, stirring to wilt as you go, until all the spinach is incorporated. It may look like a lot but it will cook down quite a bit. Add sesame oil and sesame seeds and stir.

- Take off from the stove, garnish with the preserved green onions, and serve warm. Serve with noodles, brown rice, or anything you'd like. To taste, add more soy sauce and chili paste or flakes.

Nutritional Information

Calories: 297kcal

Carbohydrates: 12g

Protein: 22g

Fat: 17

Quinoa and Chicken Bowl

Total time: 30 minutes   Number of Servings 4

Ingredients

1 ½ cups uncooked quinoa

1 pound boneless chicken breast or tenders

2 tablespoons olive oil divided

½ teaspoon paprika

¼ teaspoon turmeric

¼ teaspoon coriander

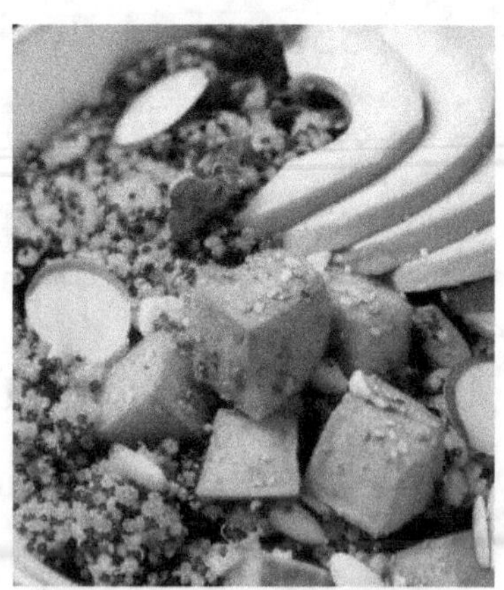

¼ teaspoon onion powder

½ teaspoon salt

¼ teaspoon black pepper

6 cups chopped kale

1 pint cherry tomatoes

½ cup toasted silvered almonds

Chopped parsley for serving

Directions

- Add 2 ¼ cups of water to a small pot with the quinoa. Over medium-high heat, bring the mixture to a boil. Reduce heat to a simmer and cook for fifteen minutes while covered. Take the saucepan off of the burner.

- Let the quinoa lie in the pot for around five minutes without lifting the cover to absorb all of the liquid and steam. Lift the lid and mix the quinoa with a fork to separate it.

- In a small bowl, combine 1 tablespoon olive oil, paprika, turmeric, coriander, onion powder, salt, and pepper. Coat the chicken with the spice mixture after adding it to the bowl.

- The remaining tablespoon of olive oil should be heated in a medium pan over medium heat. After moving the chicken to the skillet, cook it on each side for three to four minutes or until the juices run clear. Cut each breast into strips after taking it off the stove and letting it cool.

- Add the kale to the same pan you used to cook the chicken, and sauté, tossing regularly, over medium-high heat until the kale is tender and charred, 3 to 5 minutes. It might be necessary to cook in batches. Set aside.

- Add the cherry tomatoes to the same pan and sauté, turning regularly, over medium-high heat for 3 to 5 minutes or until softened and charred. Set aside.

- Place the quinoa, chicken, kale, tomatoes, and almonds in four bowls and assemble the chicken and quinoa bowls. Add some chopped parsley as a garnish, then serve right away.

Nutritional Information

Calories: 447kca

Carbohydrates: 58g

Protein: 17g

Fat: 19g

Grilled Portobello Mushroom Burgers

Total time: 1 hr   Number of Servings 3 −4

Ingredients

4 Portobello mushroom caps

2 tbsp. balsamic vinegar

1 tbsp. Low-sodium soy sauce

1 tablespoon olive oil

1 tbsp. chopped rosemary

1-1/2 tsp. steak seasoning like Montreal Steak Grill Mates

4 thick slices of red onion

4 oz reduced-fat Swiss, sliced thin

4 thin slices of tomato

1/2 avocado, sliced thin

Baby spinach

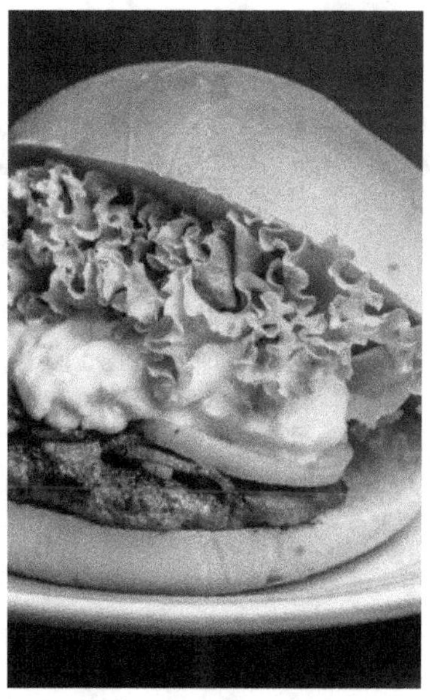

4 whole wheat low-calorie buns (I used Martin)

Directions

- Mix the oil, soy sauce, vinegar, rosemary, and Montreal steak seasoning in a big bowl.

- Toss the mushroom caps in the basin with the sauce, ensuring they are equally coated using a spoon. After a few turns, let stand at room temperature for 20 to 30 minutes.

- On medium heat, preheat the grill or indoor grill pan. Apply a little layer of oil to the grill pan or grate while it's hot.

- With the marinade reserved for basting, place the mushrooms on the grill. Grill until tender, 5 to 7 minutes per side, brushing often with marinade.

- Top the mushrooms with cheese during the last minute of cooking.

- As the mushrooms cook, toast the buns and grill the onions for approximately a minute on each side.

- Finally, top the buns with the grilled onions, sliced tomato, and avocado after adding the spinach and Portobello mushrooms.

Nutritional Information

Calories: 295 kcal

Carbohydrates: 31 g

Protein: 21 g

Fat: 13 g

Stuffed Roasted Peppers with Lentils, Beef and Mushrooms

Total time: 25 minutes   Number of Servings: 6

Ingredients

2 tbsps. Olive oil

1 pound ground beef

1/2 onion, chopped

2 cloves garlic, minced

8 mushrooms, cremini or white button; chopped

1 cup lentils, dried

2 cans tomatoes, diced, with juice (29 oz)

1/2 - 1 tsp red pepper flakes (add more for heat)

Salt and pepper

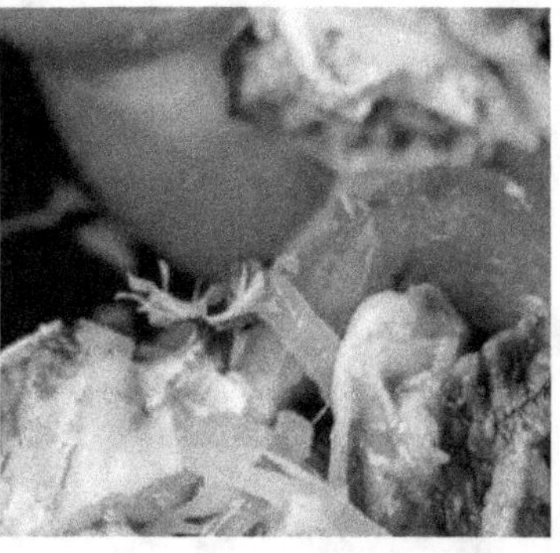

6 bell peppers, tops removed and scooped out

1 cup queso fresco (or cheese of choice)

1/2 cup cilantro, chopped

Directions

- Set the oven's temperature to 350.

- Place 3 cups of boiling water and the rinsed dry lentils in a medium-sized saucepan.

- For 20 minutes, simmer. Drain and allow to cool.

- Heat the olive oil in a big skillet. Add the garlic, onions, and a dash of salt. Simmer for 3–4 minutes or until the vegetables start to soften. Then, add the mushrooms and simmer for 5–7 minutes or until tender. Take out of the skillet and transfer the onion-mushroom mixture to a bowl.

- Add the ground beef to the same skillet, season with salt, and cook until browned. Add the tomato paste, diced tomatoes with juice, and red pepper flakes and stir. Combine and let simmer for five minutes. Add the cooked lentils and the onion-mushroom combination. Add salt and pepper to taste, then adjust the spices.

- Bell peppers should be put in a big baking dish. Fill the bell peppers to the brim with the filling. Put in the oven, then roast for twenty-five minutes. After taking the peppers out of the oven, sprinkle fresh cilantro and queso fresco.

Nutritional Information

Calories: 320

Carbohydrates: 22g

Protein: 25g

Fat: 15g

Chickpea and Spinach Curry

Total time: 15 minutes   Number of Servings: 4

Ingredients

Basmati rice, to serve

Squeeze lemon juice

250g bag baby leaf spinach

2 x 400g cans chickpeas, drained and rinsed

400g can cherry tomatoes

1 onion, chopped

2 tbsp. Mild curry paste

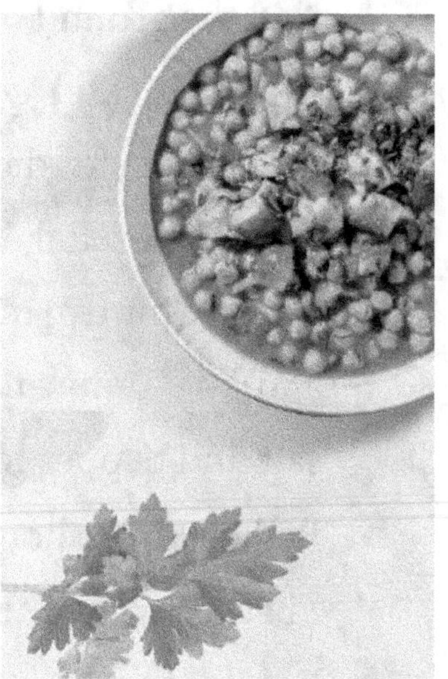

Directions

- Put the curry paste in a big, nonstick skillet and heat it. Add the onion and cook for 2 minutes to soften it. Once it splits, Add the tomatoes and let them bubble for five minutes or until the sauce thickens.

- Cook for an additional minute after adding the chickpeas and some seasoning. Turn off the heat and add the spinach, letting the pan's heat wilt the leaves. Serve with basmati rice after seasoning and adding the lemon juice.

Nutritional Information

Calories: 350

Carbohydrates: 35g

Protein: 12g

Fat: 20g

Roasted Chickpeas

Total time: 60 mins   Number of Servings: 4-6

Ingredients

2 (15-ounce) cans chickpeas

1 tablespoon olive oil

1 tablespoon ground sumac

2 teaspoons smoked paprika

1 teaspoon garlic powder

1/2 teaspoon fine sea salt

1/4 teaspoon black pepper

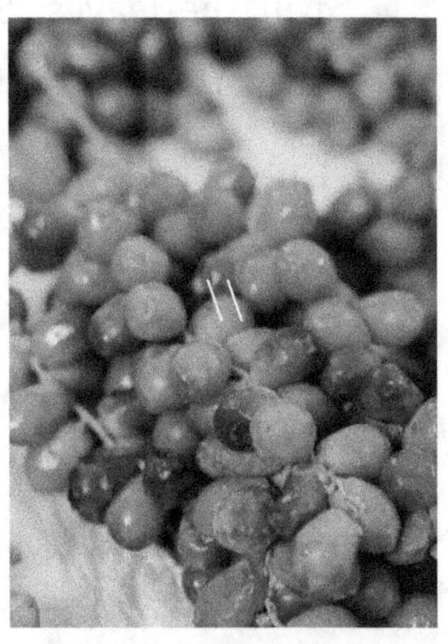

Directions

- Set up the baking sheet and oven. Adjust the oven to 350°F. Put parchment paper on the bottom of a large baking sheet.

- Dry, rinse, and drain the chickpeas. In a colander, thoroughly rinse the chickpeas until the water runs clear and they are no longer frothy. Drain completely. Lay out the chickpeas on a fresh towel, then gently wipe the chickpeas with the towel to remove as much moisture as possible. Toss away any skins that come off during the drying process.

- Season. Move the chickpeas to a generously sized mixing basin. Evenly drizzle with olive oil, add sumac, smoked paprika, garlic powder, salt, and pepper. Gently mix to coat evenly.

- Bake. Arrange the chickpeas on the prepared baking sheet in an equal layer. Bake the chickpeas for 45 minutes, shaking the pan once at the 15 and 30-minute marks or until they are crispy and dry to the touch. (However, kindly be aware that they will continue to crisp up even more after baking.)

- Serve. Serve immediately, or refrigerate at room temperature for up to three days in an uncovered jar or dish (loosely covered with a paper towel or thin kitchen towel).

Nutritional Information

Calories: 115

Carbohydrates: 12g

Protein: 6g

Fat: 3g

Trail Mix with Nuts and Seeds

Total time: 8 minutes   Number of Servings: 8

Ingredients

2 ounces unsweetened coconut flakes

4 – 8 ounces (~½ – 1 ½ cups) seeds

12-ounce bag of dark chocolate chips

Mix-ins to YOUR taste

1 pound (~3 cups) dried fruit

1 ½ pounds (~5 cups) roasted, lightly salted nuts

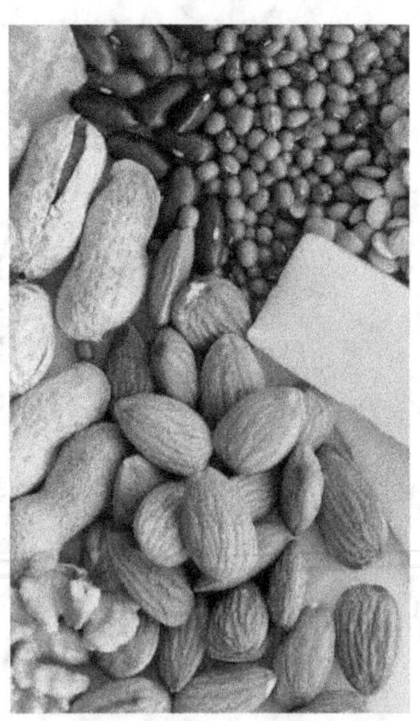

Directions

Mix the ingredients by shaking or stirring them in a big bag or container. Enjoy!

Nutritional Information

Calories: 336

Carbohydrates: 22g

Protein: 11g

Fat: 25g

Veggie Sticks with Hummus

Total time: 10 minutes   Number of Servings: 1

Ingredients

50g/3.5oz red capsicum/bell pepper (1/4 medium capsicum)

50g/1.8oz celery

100g/3.5oz carrot (abt 1 small-med size)

150g/5.3oz Homemade hummus or 75g store-bought hummus*

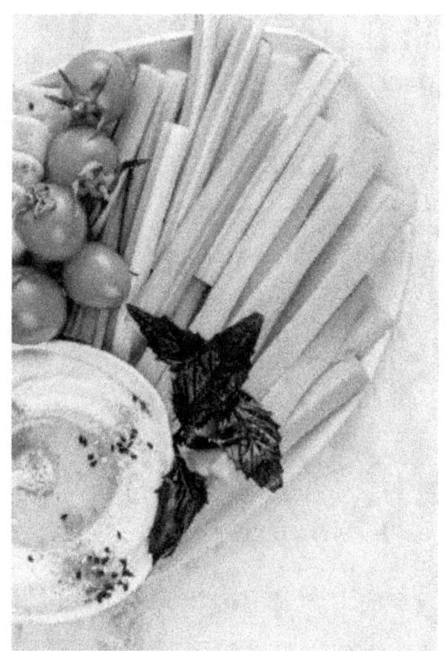

Directions

- To prepare your hummus, follow this simple method. It takes ten minutes or less.

- Thinly slice the carrot, celery, and capsicum.

- When ready to serve, arrange the hummus in a bowl and the rest of the ingredients on a platter.

Nutritional Information

Calories: 271

Carbohydrates: 27g

Protein: 16g

Fat: 11g

Homemade Fruit and Nut Bars

T/ time: 2 hrs 45 mins   N/ of Servings: 12 bars

Ingredients

1 cup honey

2 tsp vanilla extract

½ tsp salt

1 Tbsp flaxseeds

¼ cup sesame seeds

¼ cup pumpkin seeds

¼ cup sunflower seeds

½ cup dried cranberries

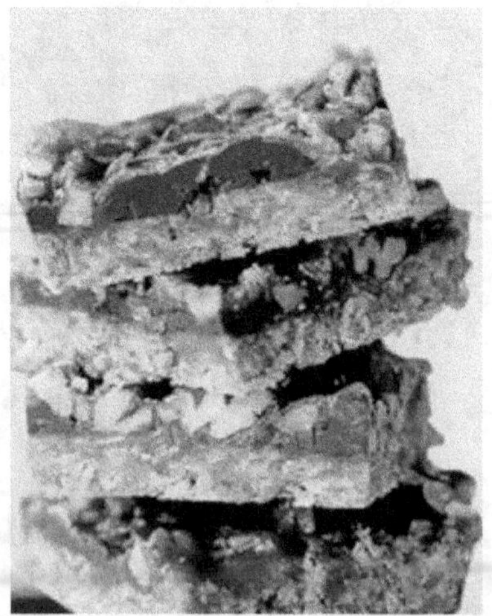

1 cup chopped nuts (use cashews, walnuts, pecans, almonds, macadamia nuts, etc.)

1 cup whole nuts (use cashews, walnuts, pecans, almonds, macadamia nuts, etc.)

Directions

- Set oven temperature to 350°F. Line an 8-inch square baking sheet with parchment paper and coat with cooking spray.

- Combine all the ingredients in a sizable bowl and thoroughly combine them.

- Spoon the batter into the baking pan. Press firmly on the nuts to flatten them into a single layer using the spatula.

- Bake the nuts for 40 to 50 minutes or until they begin to color to some extent. Their color will be a rich, deep shade of golden brown. The bars in the pan should cool fully for two to three hours. After moving to a chopping board, cut into 12 bars.

- Individually wrap each bar in parchment paper. For extended storage, freeze or refrigerate for a week.

Notes

- We use one cup of whole nuts and one cup of coarsely chopped nuts to make the mixture stick together beautifully. It's up to you to utilize all of the nuts or not.
- If you use substitutes, make sure the amounts stay the same so that everything is well coated in honey; if not, the ingredients won't stick to one another.
- Put parchment paper on the baking pan for easy removal and cleanup.
- Once the nut and seed mixture is on the baking sheet, cover it with a layer of parchment paper that has been oiled and press the mixture firmly into the pan using the bottom of a strong glass.

- Run a spatula over the pan's edges when ready to remove the bars.

- Divide the bars into twelve equal halves.

- Instead of sawing, use a sharp knife and pressure to cut.

- To keep the bars fresh, wrap them in parchment paper.

Nutritional Information

Calories: 242kcal

Carbohydrates: 22g

Protein: 5g

Fat: 17g

Smoothie Packs

Total time: 5 minutes   Number of Servings: 8

Ingredients

100 g (3.33 cups) Spinach

400 g (2.75 cups) Strawberries - hulled and halved

200 g (1.66 cups) raspberries

200 g (1.33 cups) Blueberries

4 Banana - cut into chunks

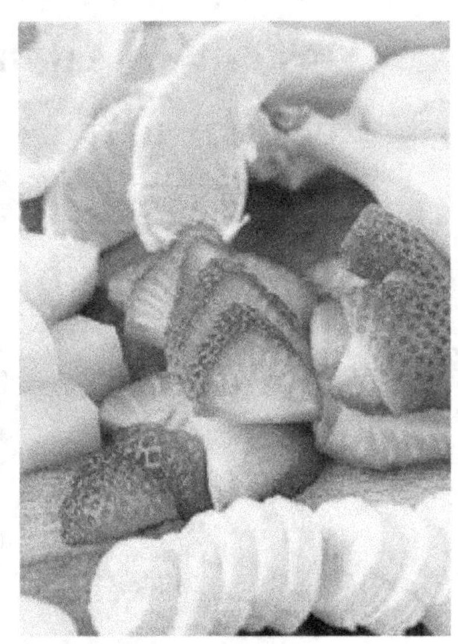

Directions

- Put spinach in a Ziploc bag or something similar.

- Following that with banana chunks. Next strawberries,

- The blueberries and raspberries come last.

- Recipe tips

- Do you not like bananas? An avocado can be used in its place, which adds a creamy texture. However, it doesn't mix as well as bananas.

- Use high-quality zip-lock freezer bags, wash them after use, and store them away.

- The components can also be kept in the freezer in mason jars. Though we like bags since they can be stacked and lie flat in the freezer, they take up much more room.

- Smoothie bags will fit into the freezer more compactly if you flatten them and eliminate the air before sealing them.

- Label every smoothie bag so you know exactly when it was placed in the freezer and how long it will remain fresh.

- Your preferred smoothie consistency will determine how much liquid you put in the blender. Add as much or as little as you like.

- Four smoothie bags (two adult servings per pack) are made using this recipe. Four children who enjoy smoothies can split each bag.

Nutritional Information

Calories: 99kcal

Carbohydrates: 24g

Protein: 2g

Fat: 1g

Chia Seed Pudding

Total time: 1 hrs. 10 mins   Number of Servings: 2

Ingredients

1 cup almond milk

4 tablespoons chia seeds

*½ tablespoon maple syrup, honey, or sweetener of choice**

¼ teaspoon vanilla extract (optional)

Toppings: fresh berries or other fruit, granola, nut butter, etc.

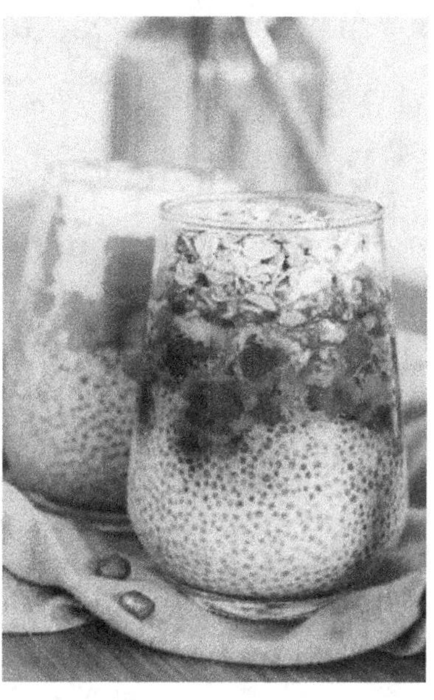

Directions

- If desired, combine the chia seeds, milk, maple syrup, and vanilla extract in a Mason jar or dish. Cover the Mason jar and shake the mixture to ensure that everything is combined.

- After thoroughly mixing the chia pudding mixture, cover and place it in the refrigerator to "set" for one to two hours or overnight. After letting it rest for five minutes, give it another toss or shake to break up any clumps of chia seeds. Instead of being runny, the chia pudding should be lovely and thick.

- Add chia seeds (approximately 1 Tablespoon), mix, and chill for a half hour if it's still too thin.
- Chia pudding keeps well in the refrigerator for up to five to seven days when kept in an airtight container.

Notes

- Meal prep: If it's more convenient, prepare your custard the night before and refrigerate it overnight. When ready to serve, sprinkle berries over the custard and dig in.
- Milk option: You may use any milk on hand, but I prefer almond milk. A creamy, light chia pudding can be made with cashew, almond, or dairy milk. A thick and rich pudding may be made with canned coconut milk.

- Low sugar: You may use stevia or monk fruit as a sugar alternative or omit the sweetener entirely for a reduced sugar version.

Nutritional Information

Calories: 170kcal

Carbohydrates: 16g

Protein: 7g

Fat: 9g

Baked Apples with Cinnamon

Total time: 1 hr. 10 mins   Number of Servings: 6

Ingredients

APPLES

6-7 medium to large apples (2 tarts like granny smith, four sweet like honey crisp // amount as original recipe is written // organic when possible)

2 tbsp. lemon juice

1 tbsp. Coconut oil (optional)

1 ½ tsps. Ground cinnamon

1 pinch nutmeg

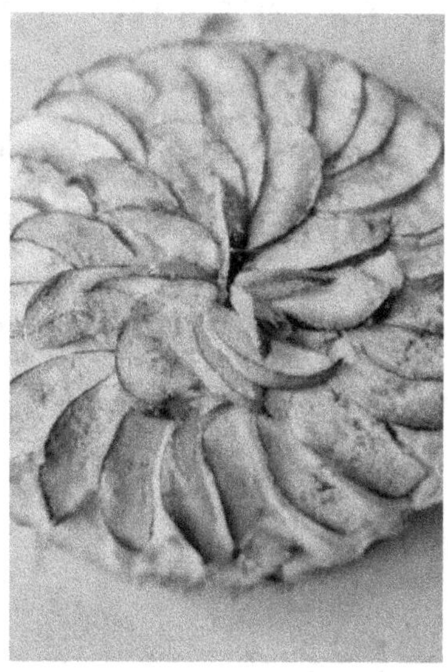

2/3 cup coconut sugar (or sub organic cane sugar // sub up to half with stevia to taste)*

*3/4 tsps. Freshly grated ginger**

3 tbsp. Cornstarch or arrowroot starch (for thickening the sauce)

3 tbsp. Fresh apple juice or water

1 pinch of sea salt

FOR SERVING (optional):

Coconut Whipped Cream

*Vanilla Bean Coconut Ice Cream*3 tbsp. Fresh apple juice or water*

1 pinch of sea salt

Directions

- Set aside a 9x13-inch (or comparable) baking dish and preheat the oven to 350 degrees Fahrenheit (176 degrees Celsius).

- Apples should be peeled, cored, and thinly sliced lengthwise with a paring knife (see photo). The ideal weight is reduced! Just make an effort to cook them consistently.

- Transfer to a baking dish, then drizzle with the following ingredients: apple juice (or water), cinnamon, ginger, nutmeg, coconut sugar, coconut oil (optional), and a generous amount of salt. To mix, toss. After that, wrap loosely with foil.

- Bake, covered, for 45 minutes. After that, gently take off the foil and bake for 10 to 15 minutes, or until the apples are very soft to the fork and have started to caramelize somewhat in the middle of the dish.

- Savor it alone or pair it with Vanilla Bean Coconut Ice Cream or Coconut Whipped Cream! Although leftovers can be frozen for up to a month or kept covered in the refrigerator for up to four days, they are best when fresh.

- Warm the food again in a microwave or a covered oven set at 350 degrees Fahrenheit (176 degrees Celsius). Add a small amount of water if the "caramel" sauce is too thick.

Nutritional Information

Calories: 195

Carbohydrates: 50.6 g

Protein: 0.3 g

Fat: 0.2 g

Avocado Chocolate Mousse

Total time: 1 hr. 10 mins   Number of Servings: 4

Ingredients

Whipped cream for serving

Raspberries for serving

Pinch sea salt

2 teaspoons vanilla extract

2 tablespoons maple syrup

¼ cup almond milk

¼ cup cocoa powder

½ cup bittersweet chocolate bar melted

2 very ripe avocados

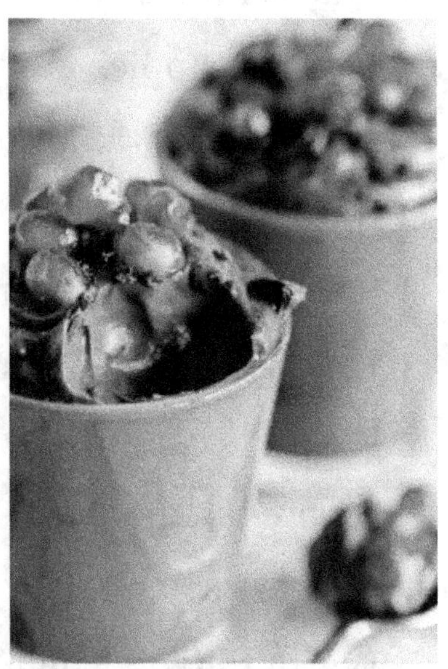

Directions

- Add the avocados, almond milk, melted chocolate, cocoa powder, vanilla extract, maple syrup, and salt to a food processor or high-speed blender. Stir until creamy and smooth, approximately 2 minutes; scrape down sides as necessary.

- To make the mousse more mousse-like, divide it evenly among four dishes or jars and refrigerate for at least an hour.
- Top the mousse with coconut whipped cream and raspberries, and serve cool if preferred.

Nutritional Information

Calories: 335kcal

Carbohydrates: 30g

Protein: 4g

Fat: 24g

Oatmeal Banana Cookies

T/ time: 20 mins   Numb of Servings: 18 Cookies

Ingredients

3 bananas, overripe (about 1 ¼ cups mashed banana)

2 tablespoons honey (or maple syrup)

1 egg

1 teaspoon pure vanilla extract

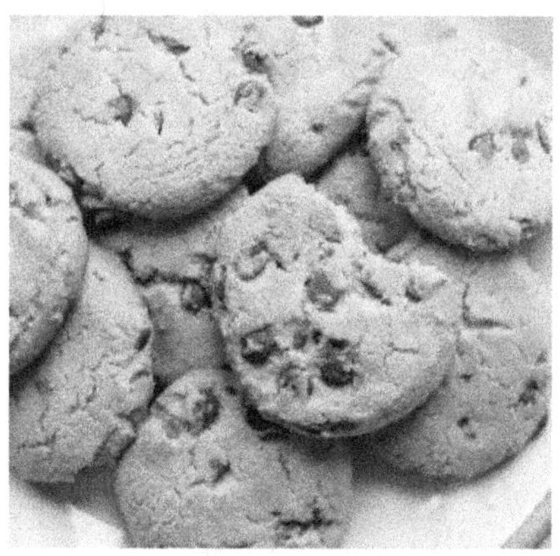

1 ½ cups quick-cooking oats

1 teaspoon ground cinnamon

¼ teaspoon fine sea salt

½ cup chocolate chips or other add-ins like shredded coconut, dried cranberries, raisins, etc.

Directions

- Set oven temperature to 350°F. Put parchment paper on two baking sheets and set them aside.

- Mash the bananas in a large mixing dish.

- Stir together the egg, vanilla, and honey.

- Stir together the sea salt, cinnamon, and oats.

- Stir in mix-ins until they are spread evenly, if desired.

- Spoon approximately 2 inches apart on the prepared baking sheet, scooping out parts of the dough using a 1 tablespoon measuring spoon or a 1 ½ TBS cookie scoop.

- Bake for 12 to 15 minutes until the bottoms are lightly browned and the tops are set. The oven should be warmed.
- Allow to cool on the baking sheet for five minutes, then move to a wire cooling rack to cool entirely.
- Warm or room temperature serving is recommended.

Notes

To store or freeze:

Keep in an airtight container for two days at room temperature, five to seven days in the fridge, or two months in the freezer.

Ingredient Substitutions

- ripe bananas. Verify that the bananas you have are sweet and ripe. If you are using frozen bananas, defrost them in the microwave or at room temperature before using them in this recipe.

- Maple syrup with honey. Each liquid sweetener is effective. You may also use brown rice syrup or agave nectar.

- Egg. To make them vegan or egg-free, use a flax or egg substitute.

- Quick-cooking oats. You can use old-fashioned or rolled oats, but the texture will differ.

- Cinnamon. Don't overlook it! These are the finest banana oatmeal cookies ever, thanks to the cinnamon.

- Sea salt. Cut in half if you're using iodized salt.

- Chocolate chips. In this recipe, regular-sized or microchips work nicely. Additional options include chopped nuts, peanut butter chips, coconut, raisins, cherries, cranberries, blueberries, and other dried fruit. White chocolate chips, coconut, and chopped almonds are all options.

Nutritional Information

Calories: 79kcal

Carbohydrates: 15g

Protein: 2g

Fat: 2g

Frozen Berry Sorbet

Total time: 1 hrs.   Number of Servings: 4

Ingredients

SYRUP

1 cup water

2/3 cup sugar

SMOOTHIE BASE

1 cup frozen strawberries

2/3 cup frozen blueberries

1/4 cup lemon juice

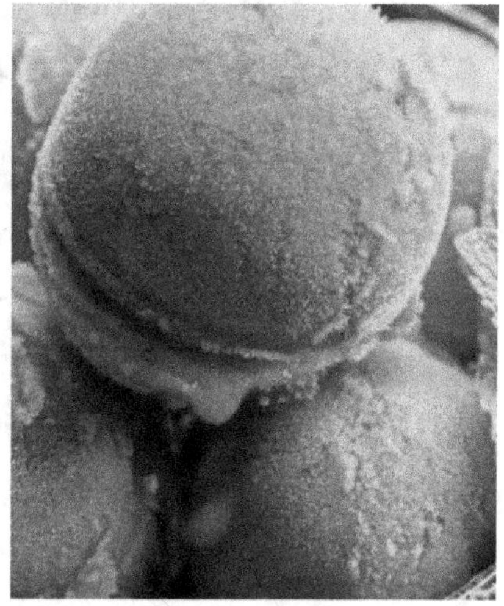

Directions

- Combine the sugar and water in a small pot to prepare the syrup. Heat gently over medium heat, stirring until sugar dissolves completely. Remove from heat. The syrup doesn't need to be boiled; it will cool down more quickly the less heat it receives.

- It's time to prepare the sorbet once the syrup has cooled down enough that you can easily insert your finger into it without discomfort.

- Fill the blender with blueberries first, then strawberries. Incorporate the lemon juice and sufficient syrup to submerge the berries partially. Blend, pulse, and so on until the puree is smooth. Serve immediately or, to avoid freezer burn, freeze in a plastic jar with a layer of wax paper or saran wrap touching the top. Take it out of the freezer five to ten minutes before serving so it can soften.

Nutritional Information

Calories: 100

Carbohydrates: 23g

Protein: 2g

Fat: 0g

CHAPTER TWELVE

Strong evidence suggests that one of the most effective strategies for preventing cancer may be consuming a plant-based diet high in fruits, vegetables, whole grains, and legumes. Because of their high fiber content, high antioxidant and anti-inflammatory chemical levels, and other factors, these dietary categories have been linked to a considerably decreased risk of cancer.

Insulin resistance, hormone/growth factor dysregulation, oxidative stress, inflammation, exposure to carcinogens, and an unhealthy gut microbiome are among the risk factors that, if uncontrolled, encourage cancer development. Plant-based diets help lessen these risks.

Eating a diet high in fruits, vegetables, whole grains, seeds, nuts, and legumes encourages our gut microorganisms to make butyrate, a kind of short-chain fatty acid that has been found to reduce inflammation and even prevent the growth of colon cancer.

According to in-depth research published in the International Journal of Cancer, eating a diet high in plant foods and low in animal foods lowered cancer risk by fifteen percent.

Over 34 years, a prominent Harvard study examined whether participants followed five low-risk lifestyle factors: never smoking, maintaining a healthy weight, exercising frequently, consuming alcohol in moderation, and adhering to a healthy diet rich in fruits, vegetables, whole grains, unsaturated fats, and omega-3 fats and low in trans fats, red and processed meats, and sugar-sweetened beverages. Researchers discovered that only maintaining a nutritious diet lowered the chance of dying from cancer by thirty percent; maintaining all five of these healthy lifestyle characteristics reduced the risk of dying from cancer by sixty-five percent.

Antioxidant-Rich Foods and Their Cancer-Preventing Benefit

Eating a low-fat diet high in veggies and whole grains has been shown in studies to help increase cancer patient's chances of survival. Research has demonstrated an 18% reduction in the probability of dying from colorectal cancer, including 1,575 individuals who did not have metastatic colorectal cancer for every 5 grams of increased daily fiber consumption. (The sole sources of fiber are plant foods; animal products don't contain any fiber.) In research examining the relationship between food and mortality from breast cancer, women who ate more fruits, vegetables, and whole grains also lived longer. The possibility that some plant-based diets might inhibit angiogenesis—the process by which our bodies form new blood vessels, which cancer cells can exploit to increase and spread—is one topic of ongoing research.

CHAPTER THIRTEEN

Holistic Approach to Health

Optimal health and surviving cancer

Those undergoing cancer treatment embark on a new chapter that may have excitement, anxiety, optimism, and happiness. No two people are alike. Everybody copes and learns to control these emotions differently. It will require practice and time.

You may find yourself contemplating death and dying, and you may be worried that the cancer may return. Cancer survivors frequently have a dread of cancer returning, also known as cancer recurrence, which can occasionally be extremely strong.

You may be more conscious of how the disease has affected your friends, family, and professional life. You could examine your interactions with people in your immediate vicinity in a fresh light. Unexpected problems might also be problematic. For example, you may be anxious about money due to your medical care. After treatment, you may also have more free time and see your medical team less frequently. You may feel nervous about any of these things.

For life after cancer, some people are more equipped than others. However, assistance and support from others—whether from friends and family, religious organizations, support groups, licensed counselors, or others—can benefit everyone.

You have been visiting your cancer care team often, but suddenly, you are not required to go for several months at a time. Some patients believe they are no longer fighting the disease after therapy. Anxiety may arise. You may feel lost and alone without your cancer care team's assistance. These folks could now play a significant role in your life. You might feel depressed and worried not to see them.

Resuming your place in the family may also prove to be more difficult than you anticipated. The things that you used to accomplish are now being done by others because of your sickness. Perhaps they are unwilling to return your responsibilities to you. You may have an issue with someone else's approach but are hesitant to voice your disagreement.

Some patients experience overwhelming grief, rage, or terror when feelings they've suppressed during cancer treatment suddenly resurface. Some of it could be the residual effects of your medication, but other times, it seems like your body and soul are worn out and need a protracted nap. It's been a while since you were able to unwind.

These emotions all make sense. You recently went through a trying period. You've had to make some significant choices in life. Cancer has attacked your body, and so has its therapy. For a while at least, your whole perspective and manner of living have evolved.

It is crucial to acknowledge these emotions and develop coping mechanisms for them. Thinking things will return as they were before your diagnosis is unrealistic. Allow time to pass; you, your loved ones, and others in your immediate vicinity will overcome this. You can get used to life after cancer, just as it took some time to get used to cancer.

Remaining optimistic

A lot of focus has been placed on maintaining a positive outlook in recent years. Some even claim that adopting such a mindset will prevent the disease from spreading or from returning. Please do not let this load be placed on you by the mistaken attempts of others to promote positive thinking.

If you can see the bright side of things, you might be able to handle your life and cancer history more effectively, but that's not always feasible. It's beneficial to strive for a positive outlook since it might make you feel better about your current situation in life. Remember that you don't always have to project a "positive" attitude. When you're upset, depressed, furious, or nervous, don't punish yourself or allow others to make you feel bad about it.

A person's beliefs or poor attitude do not cause cancer, nor does it worsen it. Don't allow the myths about having a positive attitude outlook to prevent you from communicating your feelings to your cancer care team or loved ones.

Adjusting to a life of uncertainty

You may notice that you're focusing a lot of attention on your body's aches and pains. Feeling like a "sitting duck" is possible. You say you don't have any cancerous indications right now, but are you sure? One may wonder...

Will it return?

What are the odds that it will return?

How can I tell if it has returned?

How would I respond if it reappears?

When is it going to return?

You get terrified and find it difficult to sleep, spend quality time with your partner, or make straightforward judgments. It is not just you.

Many people report that as time passes, they find themselves thinking about cancer less and less and that their dread of cancer coming back (recurrence) diminishes. However, some situations may rekindle this concern years after therapy, such as a

Visits for follow-up or specific medical testing

Dates of anniversaries (such as the day you received a diagnosis, underwent surgery, or finished treatment)

On birthdays

Illness of a relative

Finding out that a loved one has cancer or has experienced a relapse

Experiencing symptoms that have a striking resemblance to your initial cancer diagnosis

Novel symptoms that you don't comprehend

The passing of a cancer patient

The following suggestions have assisted others in overcoming anxiety and uncertainty and feeling more hopeful:

Know your stuff. Find more about the resources available to you and what you can do right now to improve your health. Your sensation of control may increase as a result.

Recognize that you have no control over the recurrence of cancer. Instead of fighting this, it is helpful to embrace it.

Recognize your fears, but don't assign labels to them. Try letting them go a little. These kinds of ideas are common, but they don't have to stay with you. Some imagine things dissipating or disintegrating. Some give them up to a greater force to manage. Whatever method you choose, letting things go will help you avoid squandering time and effort on pointless anxiety.

Speak to a trustworthy friend or counselor about your emotions of dread or doubt. Many people find that becoming vulnerable and addressing their feelings reduces anxiety. Research has shown that expressing intense emotions like dread helps people let go of those experiences more efficiently. It might not be easy to think about and discuss your sentiments. However, finding a means to communicate your feelings might be helpful if you discover that cancer is taking over your life.

Instead of dwelling on the past or the unknown future, focus on the here and now. If you can manage to discover inner peace, even if it's just for a little while each day, you'll be able to remember that calm amid a chaotic and hectic existence.

Concentrate on your well-being and the actions you can do right now to maintain your current level of health. Try to alter your diet healthily. If you smoke, this is a perfect moment for you to give it up.

Seek out strategies for relaxing.

Try to get as much exercise as you can.

Control what you can. Some claim that becoming more organized in their lives helps them feel less afraid. Among the things you can manage are changing your lifestyle, going back to your regular routine, and participating in your healthcare. You may get greater strength even just by creating a daily regimen. Even though nobody can stop thinking, some claim to have decided to ignore their fears.

Lifestyle Changes for Long-Term Health

Strong evidence suggests that eating a diet rich in fruits and vegetables can help reduce the risk of chronic illnesses, including diabetes, heart disease, and some forms of cancer. For example, the risk of getting breast and colorectal cancers can be significantly reduced by following a balanced diet and forming healthy behaviors.

Risks

According to research, diets heavy in processed and red meats—such as lamb, cattle, hog, liver, hot dogs, and deli meat—can increase your chance of developing colorectal cancer. Furthermore, charring or extremely high cooking temperatures might produce toxic compounds that increase the risk of colorectal cancer. Drinking alcohol raises the risk of breast cancer and is also connected to colorectal cancer.

Compared to women who abstain from alcohol, those who consume two to five drinks daily are approximately 1.5 times more likely to get breast cancer. The American Cancer Society advises that women limit their daily alcohol consumption to one drink. Twelve ounces of standard beer, five ounces of wine, or 1.5 ounces of 80-proof distilled spirits are considered drinks.

Make an effort to consume a diet high in whole grains, low-fat dairy products, lean meats, legumes, nuts, and seeds. Polyphenols, omega-3 fatty acids, and antioxidants are among the valuable ingredients found in the majority of these meals. Super foods, also referred to as functional foods, reduce oxidative and inflammatory damage. Natural processes like oxidation cause harm to cells and tissues and may be a factor in some diseases. Research has demonstrated the genuine potential of plant-based nutrition over time and linked particular meals to a lower chance of developing certain cancers. Garlic, for instance, is a potent anti-inflammatory and may help prevent cancer, particularly colon cancer. Crushed garlic is also discovered to have higher health benefits than raw garlic.

Exercise

In addition to maintaining a healthy diet, up your physical activity level to help avoid cancer. Regular exercise has been shown in studies to lower the risk of cancer. According to one research, brisk walking for one hour and fifteen minutes to two and a half hours per week lowered a woman's risk of breast cancer by 18%. Walking for ten hours or more per week may significantly lower risk.

According to the American Cancer Society, individuals should engage in 150 minutes per week of moderate-intensity physical exercise or 75 minutes per week of vigorous-intensity physical activity (or a combination), ideally spaced out throughout the course of the week.

All the benefits of a plant-based diet will eventually become apparent via more research into foods and their functional ingredients. Until then, you may increase your chances of avoiding cancer by eating various fruits and vegetables cooked in different ways. Additionally, remember to combine a healthy diet with lots of exercise.

Conclusion

The importance of a plant-based diet in achieving optimal health and preventing cancer cannot be emphasized. As we wrap out this thorough guide, let's consider the powerful effects of switching to a plant-based diet, especially for women.

Your greatest asset is your health. Therefore, deciding to take charge of your well-being is powerful. Making decisions that align with your long-term and short-term vitality when you adopt a plant-based diet is an active aspect of your health journey.

Living a plant-based lifestyle gives a comprehensive approach to bodily nourishment in addition to a diet. It becomes a cornerstone for general well-being and transcends the immediate objective of cancer prevention. You are embracing a world of nutrient-dense, entire foods instead of merely avoiding specific meals.

Adopting a plant-based diet can be quite beneficial for women in particular. A plant-based diet is an effective weapon in a woman's health toolbox because of the complex relationship between nutrition and hormone health and the recognized connection between cancer prevention and nutrition.

This guide's chapters have uncovered the benefits of a plant-based diet in combating cancer and have highlighted the power of healthy eating. Every meal, from nutrient-dense smoothies to filling main courses and decadent yet nutrient-dense desserts, adds to a tasty and well-rounded approach to well-being.

Gaining an understanding of the significance of antioxidants and fiber gives you strength. Fiber helps to cleanse, regulate, and promote digestion; antioxidants protect cells from harm caused by free radicals. This understanding serves as your shield while you work to improve your health.

Finally, switching to a plant-based diet is a commitment to long-term health rather than only a transient alteration. It becomes a compass that leads you to a life full of vitality, vigor, and resilience beyond cancer prevention.

To maintain a holistic approach to health, remember that choosing plant-based meals is an intentional decision to support your body, mind, and soul. With plant-based nutrition, you take control of your health journey and can steer towards a future of well-being.

In conclusion, cheers to the women who begin using plant-based nourishment's transforming potential to empower themselves. I hope your path is colorful, your decisions are fulfilling, and your well-being is proof of the inner power. Cheers to embracing the limitless potential of a plant-powered existence and taking charge of your health path!

BONUS
14-DAY PLANT-BASED MEAL PLAN

DAY 1:

Breakfast: Oatmeal with Fresh Fruit

Lunch: Chickpea Crepes with Spinach and Mushroom Pesto

Dinner: Lentil and Vegetable Stir-Fry

Dessert: Apricot Pecan Bars

Snack: Roasted Chickpeas

DAY 2:

Breakfast: Scrambled Turmeric Tofu with Greens

Lunch: Zucchini Noodles with Pesto and Cherry Tomatoes

Dinner: Mushroom and Spinach Stuffed Portobello Mushrooms

Dessert: Berry Bliss Smoothie

Snack: Trail Mix with Nuts and Seeds

DAY 3:

Breakfast: Pumpkin Spice Overnight Oats

Lunch: Sweet Potato and Black Bean Enchiladas

Dinner: Quinoa Salad with Chickpeas and Lemon-Tahini Dressing

Dessert: Oatmeal Banana Cookies

Snack: Veggie Sticks with Hummus

DAY 4:

Breakfast: Sautéed Chard with Feta and Egg Breakfast Toast

Lunch: Easy Sweet Potato and Black Bean Burrito Bowls

Dinner: Oven-Roasted Brussels sprouts

Dessert: Chia Seed Pudding

Snack: Homemade Fruit and Nut Bars

DAY 5:

Breakfast: Cottage Cheese, Cucumber, and Tomato Toast

Lunch: Cauliflower and Chickpea Curry

Dinner: Stuffed Bell Peppers with Quinoa and Black Beans

Dessert: Avocado Chocolate Mousse

Snack: Smoothie Packs

DAY 6:

Breakfast: Peanut Butter Toast with Banana and Chia Seeds

Lunch: Mango and Black Bean Salad

Dinner: Roasted Butternut Squash Soup

Dessert: Frozen Berry Sorbet

Snack: Roasted Chickpeas

DAY 7:

Breakfast: Mashed Avocado Toast with Feta and Pepitas

Lunch: Quinoa Salad with Avocado and Lime Dressing

Dinner: Green Goddess Smoothie

Dessert: Blueberry Kale Elixir

Snack: Veggie Sticks with Hummus

DAY 8:

Breakfast: Refried Beans, Pico, and Sunny Side Egg Breakfast Toast

Lunch: spicy chickpea wraps with spinach and avocado

Dinner: Turmeric Lentil Soup

Dessert: Mango Matcha Smoothie

Snack: Trail Mix with Nuts and Seeds

DAY 9:

Breakfast: Bagel Avocado Toast with Salmon

Lunch: Lentil and Vegetable Stir-Fry

Dinner: Quinoa and Chicken Bowl

Dessert: Carrot Ginger Zinger Juice

Snack: Smoothie Packs

DAY 10:

Breakfast: Cabbage and Lentil Tacos with Cilantro-Lime Slaw

Lunch: Spinach, Mushroom & Pepper Stuffed Shells

Dinner: Grilled Portobello Mushroom Burgers

Dessert: Golden Glow Turmeric Smoothie

Snack: Chia Seed Pudding

DAY 11:

Breakfast: Easy Vegan Spinach & Artichoke Quiche

Lunch: spinach & chickpea curry

Dinner: Stuffed Roasted Peppers with Lentils, Beef and Mushrooms

Dessert: Blueberry Kale Elixir

Snack: Frozen Berry Sorbet

DAY 12:

Breakfast: Chickpea and Vegetable Stir-Fry

Lunch: Quinoa Salad with Chickpeas and Lemon-Tahini Dressing

Dinner: Cauliflower and Chickpea Curry

Dessert: Avocado Chocolate Mousse

Snack: Veggie Sticks with Hummus

DAY 13:

Breakfast: Spaghetti with Lentil Bolognese

Lunch: Chickpea and Spinach Curry

Dinner: Mushroom and Spinach Stuffed Portobello Mushrooms

Dessert: Berry Bliss Smoothie

Snack: Homemade Fruit and Nut Bars

DAY 14:

Breakfast: Oatmeal with Fresh Fruit

Lunch: Roasted Veggie and Hummus Wrap

Dinner: Stir-Fried Tofu with Broccoli and Teriyaki Sauce

Dessert: Frozen Berry Sorbet

Snack: Trail Mix with Nuts and Seeds

MEAL PLANNER

SHOPPING	
1	
2	
3	
4	
5	
6	
7	
8	
9	
10	
11	
12	
13	
14	
15	
16	
17	
18	
19	
20	
12	
22	
23	
24	
25	
26	
27	
28	
29	
30	
31	
32	
33	
34	
35	

MONDEY

BREAKFAST	
LUNCH	
DINNER	
SNACKS	

TUESDAY

BREAKFAST	
LUNCH	
DINNER	
SNACKS	

WEDNESDAY

BREAKFAST	
LUNCH	
DINNER	
SNACKS	

THURSDAY

BREAKFAST	
LUNCH	
DINNER	
SNACKS	

FRIDAY

BREAKFAST	
LUNCH	
DINNER	
SNACKS	

SATURDAY

BREAKFAST	
LUNCH	
DINNER	
SNACKS	

SUNDAY

BREAKFAST	
LUNCH	
DINNER	
SNACKS	

MEAL PLANNER

MONDEY	
BREAKFAST	
LUNCH	
DINNER	
SNACKS	
TUESDAY	
BREAKFAST	
LUNCH	
DINNER	
SNACKS	
WEDNESDAY	
BREAKFAST	
LUNCH	
DINNER	
SNACKS	
THURSDAY	
BREAKFAST	
LUNCH	
DINNER	
SNACKS	
FRIDAY	
BREAKFAST	
LUNCH	
DINNER	
SNACKS	
SATURDAY	
BREAKFAST	
LUNCH	
DINNER	
SNACKS	
SUNDAY	
BREAKFAST	
LUNCH	
DINNER	
SNACKS	

SHOPPING

1	
2	
3	
4	
5	
6	
7	
8	
9	
10	
11	
12	
13	
14	
15	
16	
17	
18	
19	
20	
12	
22	
23	
24	
25	
26	
27	
28	
29	
30	
31	
32	
33	
34	
35	

MEASUREMENT CONVERSION CHART

VOLUME

Unit	US	Metric
Cup	237 ml	250 ml
Teaspoon	5 ml	5 ml
Tablespoon	15 ml	15ml
Fluid ounce	29.5 ml	30 ml
Pound	454 g	450 g
Gallon	3.785 L	4L
Ounce	28.35 g	28 g

TEMPERATURE

Fahrenheit	Celsius
32°F	0°C
212°F	100°C
0°F	-17.8°C
100°F	37.8°C

Unit	Unit	Metric
Gram	1 g	1 g
Milligram	0.001 g	1 mg
Kilogram	1000 g	1 kg
Ounce	28.35 g	28 g
Pound	453.59 g	450 g